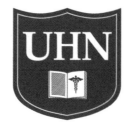

Foot & Ankle Health

Treating and Preventing Common Conditions, Ailments, and Injuries

A Special Report published
by the editors of University Health News
(www.UniversityHealthNews.com)

Foot & Ankle Health

Medical Editor: Michelle Lee, BA

Author: Jim Brown, PhD

Content Director, Belvoir Media Group: Larry Canale
Creative Director, Belvoir Media Group: Judi Crouse
Production: Karen Watson

Publisher, Belvoir Media Group: Timothy H. Cole
Executive Editor, Book Division, Belvoir Media Group: Lynn Russo Whylly

ISBN 978-1-941937-45-7

To order additional copies of this report or for customer service questions, please call 877-300-0253, or write to Health Special Reports, 535 Connecticut Avenue, Norwalk, CT 06854-1713.

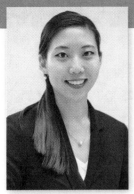

Michelle Lee, BA
(MD expected in 2019 from Weill Cornell Medical College)

Welcome to *Foot & Ankle Health*, the latest in our series of reports that deliver important health information to hundreds of thousands of people each year.

We often take the health of our feet and ankles for granted, even though they provide the support on which the rest of our bodies depend. As a result, millions of Americans seek treatment each year for problems that could be mitigated or potentially avoided.

The purpose of this report is to provide you with comprehensive, practical, and up-to-date information on foot and ankle conditions and diseases. The information reflects best practices and scientific research conducted at the leading hospitals, clinics, and institutions around the world. It includes mainstream, complementary, and integrative medical approaches.

This report also includes New Findings—brief, reader-friendly research summaries—along with concise descriptions of 38 foot and ankle disorders, 15 illustrated exercises, a glossary of 55 relevant terms, and contact information for 16 organizations and institutions.

If you're having a foot or ankle problem or you're caring for someone who does, take charge of your health-care team. Work with a primary care physician, podiatrist, orthopaedic surgeon, or other health care professional to find a long-term solution to the problem. The sooner you take action, the more likely you are to prevent a crisis later on.

We want you to make wise decisions regarding your health care, and we hope *Foot & Ankle Health* will be a step in that direction.

Sincerely,

Michelle Lee
Medical Editor

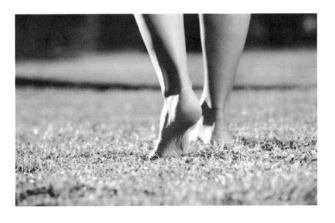

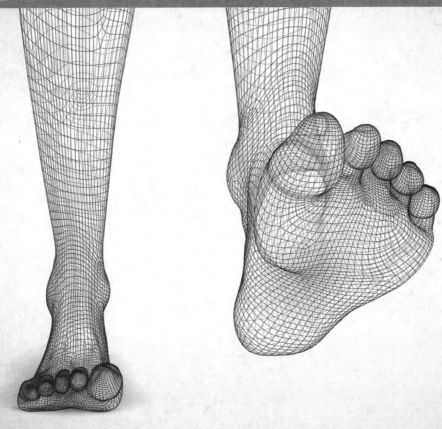

© Coffeemill | Dreamstime

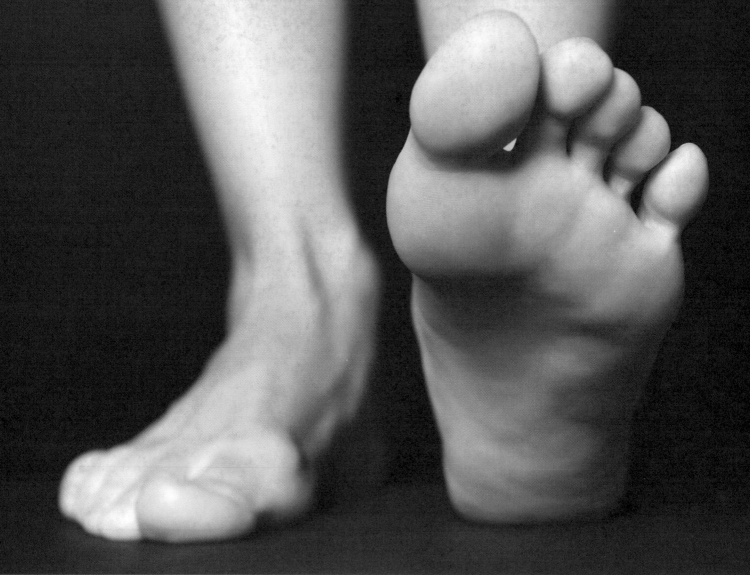

Feet can be bruised, broken, stretched, strained, and sprained, and they can be subject to diseases and inflammation like arthritis and tendinitis. One out of every 10 bones broken is in the foot. Feet can take normal, everyday wear and tear, but not overuse or neglect.

**The Feet:
By the Numbers**

- 19 muscles and tendons
- 26 bones
- 33 joints
- 107 ligaments
- 8,000 nerves
- 250,000 sweat glands

1 Foot and Ankle 101

Feet and ankles are complex, strong, and durable, but not perfect or invulnerable. Your two feet may not be the same size. They get wider and longer when we stand up and can become larger than normal at the end of a day. Some people have feet with high arches, while others are flat-footed. The ankle is one of the body's most frequently sprained joints.

The ankles are equally strong and stable, which allows them to withstand 1½ times our body weight when we walk and up to eight times when we jog or run.

The upper part of the ankle is made up of three relatively familiar bones that connect the foot to the leg: the shin bone (tibia), the calf bone (fibula), and the ankle bone (talus). Because the lower ankle is more stable than the upper ankle, injuries such as strains, sprains, and fractures nearly always affect the upper ankle.

The journal *Sports Medicine* reported that a lateral ankle sprain (outside part of joint) was the most commonly observed type of ankle sprain and that women are at higher risk than men. Other studies have shown that one of the most accurate predictors of a future ankle sprain is a past ankle sprain.

Right Up the Kinetic Chain

Doctors at the Hospital for Special Surgery (HSS) explain that the interaction between the knee and the foot, or the hip and the foot is very important because it is part of a kinetic chain. The kinetic chain means that the body's joints and segments have an effect on one another during movement and can play a key role in pain.

The foot is the first part of the body that makes contact with the ground. Its primary function is as a shock absorber. If the shock-absorbing capability of the foot is somehow altered or minimized, it's going to affect other body parts.

The foot is also the foundation of the body, say the HSS physicians. If the foundation is not sound, it could have a deleterious effect on the joints above the foot and ankle—namely the knee and the hip. Studies suggest that plantar heel pain (plantar fasciitis) may be associated with pain in the lower back.

Taking Feet for Granted

In spite of the demands we place on our feet and ankles, and despite their anatomical intricacies, we often take them for granted.

Some 75 percent of Americans will experience foot problems at least once in their lives. Our feet are spreading as they try to support the extra weight that 66 percent of Americans carry.

Nine out of 10 women wear shoes that are too small, and more than half of American women have bunions. And men can be strangely reluctant to take care of their feet.

One survey found that 28 percent of men don't even wash their feet daily. Perhaps that's why they're four times more likely to have athlete's foot than women.

What Can Go Wrong?

As already mentioned, your feet and ankles can attract a frightening array of diseases, and they can develop almost as many painful non-disease conditions. The "Causes of Foot Pain" sidebar provides a more comprehensive list of common ailments.

One of the most common causes of foot pain is not a disease, a deformity, or an injury. It's shoes: those that are too tight or too loose, that don't provide

lateral support or arch support, and that don't cushion your feet. Also, shoes with high heels, or shoes that slip on the floor, increase the risk of falls.

At-Home Treatment

Many of the problems causing foot or ankle pain can be treated at home. Throughout this report, you'll see references to the RICE protocol for pain, swelling, and inflammation.

Causes of Foot Pain		
DEFORMITIES/ BIOMECHANICAL CONDITIONS	**DISEASES/INFECTIONS/ INFLAMMATORY CONDITIONS**	**INJURIES/ TRAUMA**
• Bone spurs	• Arthritis	• Blisters
• Bunions	• Athlete's foot	• Bruises (Contusions)
• Claw toes	• Bursitis	• Dislocations
• Fallen arches	• Diabetes	• Fractures
• Flat feet	• Gout	• Muscle spasms, cramps
• Hammer toes	• Lupus	• Ruptured tendons
• High arches	• Neuromas	• Turf toe
• Mallet toes	• Peripheral artery disease	• Sprains
• Tight muscles	• Plantar fasciitis	• Strains
• Tight tendons	• Sesamoiditis	• Torn ligaments
	• Tendinitis	
	• Toenail fungus	

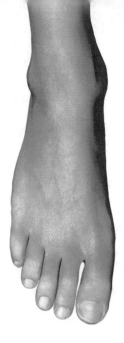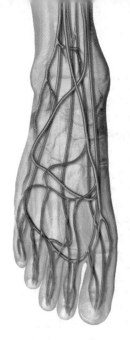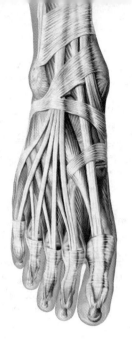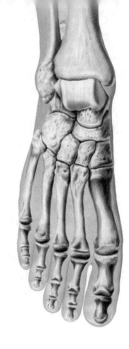

© leonello / Getty Images

Each foot is made up of 28 bones, 30 joints, and more than 100 muscles, tendons, and ligaments, all of which work together to provide support, balance, and mobility. Different authorities give different numbers in describing the anatomy of the foot, probably because some are describing the foot only, while others include the foot, ankle, and lower leg

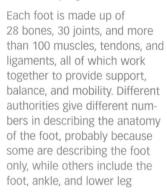

- ▶ **"R" is for REST.** Stop whatever you're doing that is causing the pain, at least until you know more about the underlying source.
- ▶ **"I" is for ICE.** Apply ice packs to the foot or ankle for 15 to 20 minutes, several times a day.
- ▶ **"C" is for COMPRESSION.** If your injury is a foot or ankle strain or sprain, wrap it tightly enough to control swelling but not so tight that it cuts off circulation.
- ▶ **"E" is for ELEVATION.** This one is not always practical, but worth trying: Elevate the affected foot or ankle at or higher than the heart to minimize swelling and control pain.

Some foot and ankle specialists add a "P" in front of the "R" (making the acronym "PRICE") when treating a muscle or joint injury:

- ▶ **"P" stands for PROTECTION, which means protect the affected area with padding, bandaging, wrapping, bracing, or splinting.**

Medications

Treatment for foot and ankle problems often involves over-the-counter (OTC) drugs and nonsteroidal anti-inflammatory drugs (NSAIDs). Some can reduce pain, some are effective at fighting inflammation, and some can do both:

- Aspirin is for pain and inflammation.

- Ibuprofen (Motrin, Advil) is for pain and inflammation.
- Naproxen (Aleve, Naprosyn) is for pain and inflammation.
- Acetaminophen (Tylenol) is for pain but not inflammation.

Check with your doctor or pharmacist before taking any new drug or a drug that might have side effects or interfere with other medications you're taking. Most are safe used for short-term relief, but each can cause problems for some people, especially if they have certain coexisting conditions.

NSAIDS like aspirin can cause bleeding in the stomach and intestines. Ibuprofen, also an NSAID, can cause stomach distress and bleeding, and should not be taken by people who have chronic kidney disease. The side effects of naproxen are upset stomach, abdominal pain, and bloating, among others. Acetaminophen is generally safe in terms of bleeding risk but can cause liver damage if taken in excessive doses.

When to See a Doctor

You should see a doctor if you notice these symptoms:

- Severe pain or swelling
- Unable to walk or put weight on your foot
- Swelling that doesn't improve after a week of home treatment

- Increased pain, redness, tenderness, or heat
- Persistent pain after two weeks
- Fever over 100°F with no apparent cause
- Burning pain, numbness, or tingling.

Which Doctor to Call

You'll have several options for getting foot and ankle care. Among the factors to take into consideration are the nature of your condition or injury (acute or chronic) and access to care—meaning proximity of the medical facility and the wait time to get an appointment. If your ankle is broken, you can't wait three weeks to see the best foot and ankle specialist in the world.

If time, circumstance, and insurance coverage allow, it's the patient's responsibility to research the expertise, credentials, and professional reputation of the doctor or other caregiver.

If you have suffered a severe injury such as a dislocation or fracture, get to an emergency room at a hospital as soon as possible. If your condition is not an emergency but serious enough to require medical attention, your choices are a walk-in, urgent-care type of facility, or your primary care doctor.

Any of those providers can give you the immediate care needed. But if the condition needs the attention of a specialist, you will be referred to either a podiatrist or an orthopaedic surgeon who specializes in the foot and ankle.

What's the Difference?

A podiatrist is a Doctor of Podiatric Medicine (DPM) who has expertise in disorders of the foot and ankle. He or she must have completed four years of undergraduate studies, four years at a podiatric medical school, and three to four years of foot and ankle surgical residency training. A podiatrist diagnoses, treats, and helps prevent foot conditions and diseases, and is likely to treat conditions conservatively before recommending surgery.

An orthopaedic surgeon is a medical doctor (MD or DO) who treats the entire musculoskeletal system, not just the foot and ankle. Training includes four years of undergraduate work, four years at a medical school, five years of surgical residency, and one year of subspecialty training to study foot and ankle disorders.

Choose the doctor with the most experience treating your condition—and one in whom you have utmost confidence.

What Happens Next?

Once you're in a doctor's care, the course of treatment is relatively predictable. It will consist of getting your medical history, a physical examination, and then x-rays, MRIs, or other imaging procedures to determine the exact nature of the condition.

Depending on the condition, your doctor may first recommend conservative (noninvasive) measures, such as physical therapy, dietary changes, lifestyle changes, weight management, foot orthotics, and medications, with surgery being a last resort.

Surgery is primarily for people with problems that cannot be successfully managed by conservative means. Examples of procedures are ankle fusion, ankle

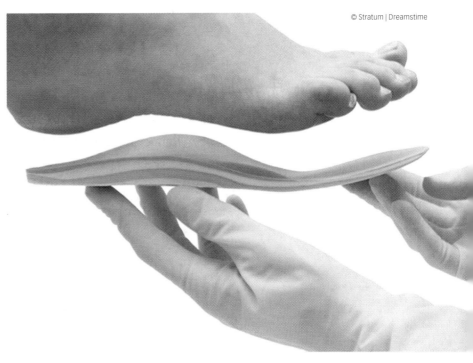

Orthopaedic insoles are designed to compensate for such issues as fallen arches.

© Stratum | Dreamstime

Soft Tissue Mobilization Effective for Heel Pain

A research team in Israel conducted a review of studies to determine whether manual therapy consisting of deep massage, myofascial release, and joint mobilization are effective in treating plantar heel pain (plantar fasciitis). Five studies showed a positive, short-term effect after manual therapy treatment, with or without stretching exercises, compared to other treatments. Moderate and high-quality studies indicated that soft tissue mobilization is an effective method for treating plantar heel pain. Outcomes for joint mobilization therapy are not conclusive.

The Foot, March 2018

replacement, tendon repair, removal of excess tissue or bone, and realignment of a bone, as well as minimally invasive treatment for plantar fasciitis, bunions, and heel spurs.

Complementary and Alternative Treatments

There is a difference between complementary treatment and alternative treatment, and it begins with an understanding of mainstream medicine. The mainstream, Western model of evidence-based medicine assumes that all medical issues can be explained in concrete terms and that the "best practice" is the result of scientific studies. Mainstream medicine uses drugs, radiation, surgery, and other methods to treat diseases and conditions.

Complementary medicine involves the use of non-mainstream practices in combination with conventional medicine. Surgery, for example, might be combined with yoga and tai chi to help regain balance.

Alternative medicine is not recognized nor endorsed by the mainstream medical community or the federal government. It is called "alternative" because it is used instead of conventional medicine.

An increasingly popular term is integrative medicine. Treatment is considered integrative when it is incorporated into mainstream, conventional care. Many major medical facilities have centers of integrative medicine, which might include acupuncture, massage therapy, or yoga, among others.

The lines between these types of medical care have begun to disappear or diminish. Some 30 percent of Americans and more than half of those over the age of 50 are using some form of medicine that is not mainstream. Acupuncture, massage, nutritional supplements, platelet-rich plasma, stem cell therapy, tai chi, and yoga are examples. Some have proven to be effective for certain conditions, some have not, and the jury is out on others.

Acupuncture

The trend has been toward more acceptance of acupuncture as a complementary treatment of certain conditions, but not necessarily foot and ankle problems. The National Center for Complementary and Integrative Health says that acupuncture appears to be a reasonable option to consider for people with chronic pain but not specifically for foot and ankle pain.

A 2017 study published in *Lasers in Medical Science* suggested that laser acupuncture might be effective for the treatment of foot pain caused by rheumatoid arthritis.

Reports suggest that the effectiveness of acupuncture varies, depending on the nature of the pain, the location, the person administering it, and the patient receiving treatment.

Laser Acupuncture May Help Rheumatoid Arthritis-Related Foot Pain

Researchers in Egypt studied the effectiveness of laser acupuncture treatment vs. reflexology in the feet and ankles as well as hands and wrists of a group of adults between 60 and 70 years of age who were diagnosed with rheumatoid arthritis. Laser acupuncture is the use of a low-level laser beam instead of an acupuncture needle to stimulate an acupuncture point. Reflexology is a therapeutic method of relieving pain by stimulating pressure points on the feet and hands.

The participants were assigned to the laser acupuncture or reflexology group. In a series of assessments of their wrists and ankles, laser acupuncture patients showed significant improvements when compared to the reflexology subjects. However, this study did not compare laser acupuncture to other rheumatoid arthritis treatments, limiting complete understanding of its efficacy.

Lasers in Medical Science, July 2017

Massage Enhances Short-Term Flexibility and Balance Functions of the Ankle

Researchers in the Republic of Korea designed a study of 32 subjects to examine the effect of calf muscle massage on ankle flexibility and balance. The participants were divided into two groups according to the massage methods applied. Both groups received five minutes of massage to each calf. Massage Group A received pressure as well as effleurage (a circular stroking movement made with the palm of the hand), and tapotement (rapid and repeating striking of the area being massaged). Group B received friction as well as effleurage and petrissage (a "kneading" type of massage).

Two tests were used to measure the results. While there was no significant differences between groups, both groups did show significant increases in balance and flexibility.

The study did not demonstrate long-term or continuing effects of massage on the two functions measured, but it suggested that massage may be helpful in short-term activities (as in a warm-up before exercise) in which balance and flexibility are needed.

Journal of Physical Therapy Science, May 2017

Massage

Therapeutic massage cannot cure or reverse the course of any disease, but it has been used by physical therapists, by massage therapists, and by patients themselves (think of rubbing an injured part of the body) for a long time. The Mayo Clinic says that massage is an effective treatment for reducing stress, pain, and muscle tension.

The evidence that massage is an effective treatment for foot and ankle disorders is limited but growing. A study in the *Journal of Physical Therapy Science* suggested that massage may be helpful in the short term for ankle flexibility and overall balance. A review of studies published in *The Foot* concluded that soft tissue manipulation is effective for treating plantar heel pain.

Chondroitin and Glucosamine

Researchers have been studying these two dietary supplements for more than two decades and the evidence is still not conclusive regarding their effects on muscle and joint pain. Most of the studies focused on knee pain, but there have been no studies on efficacy of these supplements in ankle and foot pain. Currently, the American Academy of Orthopaedic Surgeons does not recommend either supplement.

Some people use chondroitin, glucosamine, or both, and give positive anecdotal accounts. The two supplements do not appear to have negative side effects, although blood thinning is possible.

Dietary supplements fall under the Dietary Supplement Health and Education Act (DSHEA). The Food & Drug Administration (FDA) regulates dietary supplement products and ingredients under a different set of regulations than those covering foods and drugs. However, the FDA will take action against any adulterated, misbranded, or mislabeled dietary supplement.

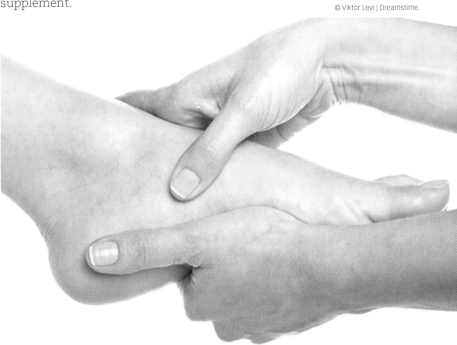

Foot massage may aid in ankle flexibility and overall balance.

© Viktor Levi | Dreamstime

Platelet-Rich Plasma

Platelet-rich plasma is derived by taking a small amount of the patient's blood, using a centrifuge to separate out the red blood cells from the whole blood, then injecting platelet-rich plasma in to the injured area.

PRP may speed up the healing and repair processes in a variety of soft-tissue injuries. It has been used to treat tendon, ligament, cartilage, and bone injuries, as well as arthritis.

Around the foot and ankle, PRP is used for treatment of tendon and ligament injuries such as plantar fasciitis, Achilles tendon, and ankle ligament injuries, according to the American Orthopaedic Foot & Ankle Society.

The position of the American Academy of Orthopaedic Surgeons (AAOS) is that while treatment with platelet-rich plasma has potential, it lacks sufficient research evidence at this point to support the claims made in the media and by clinics throughout the country.

Stem Cell Therapy

Stem cells are the body's cells grown and manipulated in a laboratory to become specific types of cells that are injected or implanted into a person. Stem cell therapy is used to promote the repair of injured tissue.

The FDA says that stem cell therapies may offer the potential to treat certain diseases or conditions and reduce inflammation, but research is still in progress. The agency warns that some patients seeking cures and remedies are vulnerable to stem cell treatments that are illegal, not-tested, and thus potentially harmful.

Peer-reviewed studies in scientific journals on stem cell therapy for foot and ankle problems are limited and inconclusive. Questions remain about timing, dosage, and effectiveness, as well as risk factors. Stem cells may be involved in some cancers, according to the Harvard Stem Cell Institute.

What Stem Cells Can Do

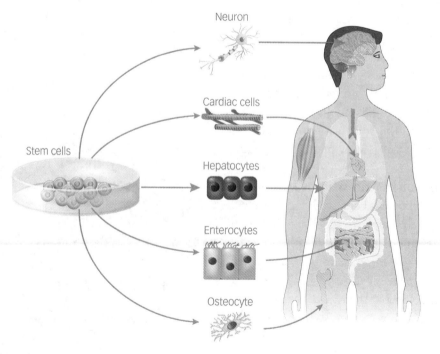

© Designua | Dreamstime

Stem cells have the potential to reduce inflammation, replicate themselves, fight cell death, and differentiate into various types of tissue.

www.universityhealthnews.com

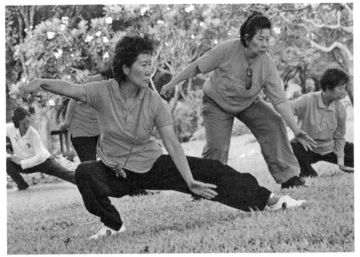
© Tuelekza | Dreamstime

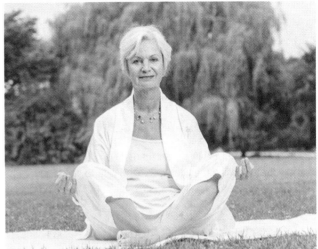
© Sureshot75 | Dreamstime

Tai Chi

Tai chi combines relaxation, meditation, and deep breathing with slow, gentle, continuous, and structured exercises.

Studies have shown that tai chi may improve balance and stability in older adults, and the National Center for Complementary and Integrative Health (NCCIH) is cautiously optimistic that it may have other benefits. Other than those regarding balance, there are no current studies on tai chi and ankle injuries or conditions.

Yoga

Yoga has been shown to relieve pain caused by several conditions, but not the feet or ankles. A study funded by the NCCIH found that people who practice yoga had significantly less pain and disability after six months. There are no specific benefits known for foot and ankle conditions.

Do tai chi (above, left) or yoga (above, right) benefit our feet and ankles? Studies haven't given such specific foot and ankle data, but research shows that tai chi provides a host of benefits (particularly balance and stability) and that yoga can result in less pain and disability.

What's Next?

Chapter 2 describes 20 orthopaedic foot and ankle conditions—how to recognize, treat, and possibly prevent them.

Shoe Fitting: A Key Step Toward Healthy Feet

If you make the mistake of buying shoes that don't fit, you'll pay twice—once at the store or online and again with problems like corns, calluses, blisters, and even sprained ankles. Our 10 tips for shoe fitting will help.

By Jim Brown, PhD, for University Health News

One of your feet may be larger than the other. Both of them change size during the day. And your feet will get bigger with age. Want to know how to handle those and related problems? Here are the answers to 10 frequently asked questions about shoe fitting.

1 What size do I ask for? You don't have to know your exact shoe size. Know your approximate size based on shoes you already own, then look for fit and comfort. Each shoe manufacturer has its own shoe size standards.

A size 9 shoe made by one company may be bigger or smaller than the same size in another brand. Trust your comfort level, not the size of a shoe. Consider tracing an outline of your foot and placing a shoe that you're considering on top of the outline. If they don't match, don't try them on.

2 When during the day should I shop for shoes? Your feet naturally swell a bit as the day wears on. Shoes that feel comfortable in the morning might feel tight in the afternoon or evening. So better to buy shoes later in the day.

3 How often should I get my feet measured? During middle-age years and beyond, it's a good idea to get your feet re-measured every year. As we age, our feet tend to get slightly larger and wider—as you've likely noticed.

4 What if one of your feet is larger than the other? It's more common than you might think. So if one of your feet is bigger than the other, the answer should be intuitive: Buy shoes that fit the larger foot. You can make up for the extra space in the smaller foot with an insert or two pairs of socks.

5 How can I tell whether my shoes are long enough? Leave room for your feet to shift forward in your shoes as you walk. Leave about a half-inch between your longest (not your big-gest) toe and the toe of the shoe. Heels should fit snugly without pinching.

6 How can I tell whether my shoes are wide enough? Shoes should be wide enough so that the widest part of your foot (the ball of the foot) is comfortable. They should also provide a comfortable degree of arch support. Also, when trying on shoes, wear the same type of socks you normally use.

7 If a shoe is too narrow, should I go up a size? Not necessarily. Look for shoes that are wider, not longer.

• For men's shoes, a narrow width is a B; a wide width is E. The average man wears a width-size D.

• Women's widths range from 4A (extra narrow) to 2E (extra wide). The average shoe width for women is B.

Shoes shouldn't have any space for your foot to move from side to side. You want "comfortably snug"—not too tight or too loose. If you're still having a shoe size problem, try another brand instead of another size.

8 How long does it take to break in a pair of shoes? No time at all. New shoes should feel comfortable the first time you put them on—not after a "break-in" period.

9 How can I test new shoes without buying them? Walk around the store on at least two different surfaces (carpet and hard floor, for example) to get a good feel. Take them

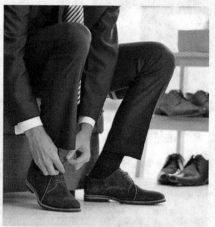

© Chernetskaya - Dreamstime

Before you buy, make sure you try on shoes, and take the time to give them a dry run. A walk around the store (on both hard flooring and carpeting, if possible) will go a long way in helping you decide whether they're the right fit.

off, put them on again, and take another lap. A test drive or two will make your decision easier.

10 What style of shoe should I avoid? This one's easy. Avoid shoes that are pointed because they crowd the toes. Women should avoid high heels in general because they put too much pressure on the forefoot. Long-term use of high heels can lead to backaches, knee pain, and sprained ankles.

More Important Than Style? Shoes That Fit

Paying attention to shoe fitting is about more than style and even comfort. It's about potential foot and toe-related problems that send 7 million Americans to the doctor every year.

Look for value, quality, and a good fit. You can get all three in one pair of shoes.

Jim Brown, PhD, is a former educator who brings a unique perspective to health and medical writing. He has authored 14 books on health, medicine, fitness, and sports.

Buying Shoes Online: If you shop for shoes online, ask about the return policy. Many companies are offering lenient terms and even encouraging customers to buy two pairs (with different sizes) to see which is better. Make sure the seller will pay for return shipping.

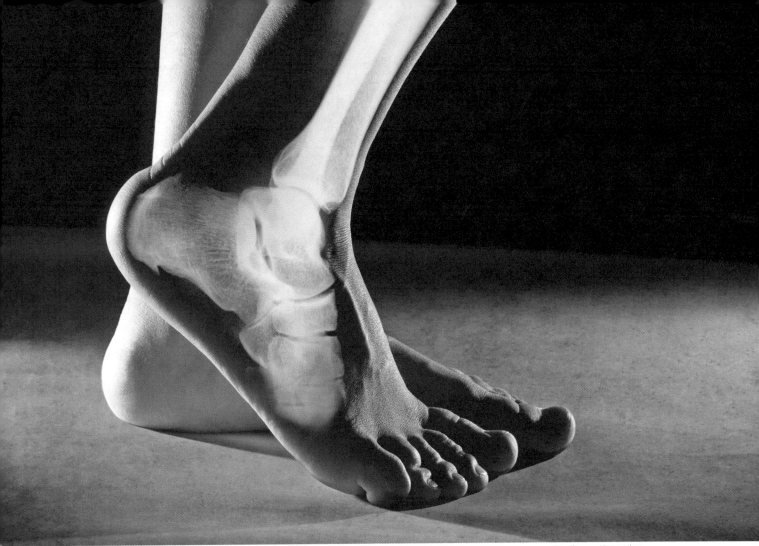

© Vadimrysev | Dreamstime

2 Orthopaedic Foot and Ankle Conditions

Highlighted in this chapter are some 21 orthopaedic foot and ankle afflictions (see index below) that make us a little—or a lot—less mobile.

Orthopaedic conditions directly involve bones, muscles, and joints. Of the 38 conditions covered in this report, 20 are orthopaedic in nature and are described in this chapter. The 17 non-orthopaedic conditions are discussed in Chapter 3.

Achilles Tendinitis

The Achilles tendon runs along the back of the lower leg, connecting the calf muscles to the heel. Without it—or without it functioning properly—we wouldn't be able to run, walk, jump, or climb stairs, among other activities. The Achilles tendon is the largest tendon in the body and can withstand a great deal of stress, but it's not invulnerable.

With natural, age-related degeneration

and/or long-term overuse, the Achilles tendon can become inflamed. The medical term is Achilles tendinitis.

Orthopaedic Foot & Ankle Conditions

Achilles Tendinitis

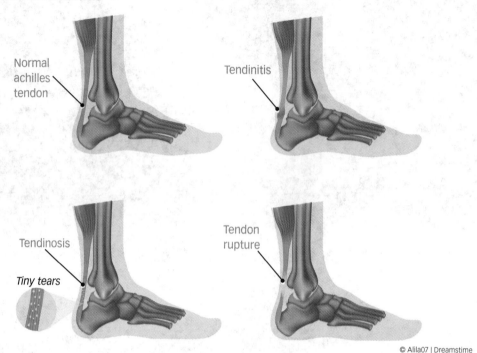

Normal achilles tendon

Tendinitis

Tendinosis

Tiny tears

Tendon rupture

© Alila07 | Dreamstime

Overuse and degeneration can cause the Achilles tendon to become inflamed, or, worse, to rupture. (*See detailed illustration of tendon rupture on page 17.*)

Symptoms

Inflammation is the way the body tries to protect itself against injury or disease, but the process involves the classic symptoms of tendinitis: pain (sometimes the day after intense exercise), swelling that becomes worse throughout the day, irritation, morning stiffness, and restricted mobility.

In younger, more active adults, tendinitis often involves the middle area of the tendon. In middle-aged and older adults, Achilles tendinitis is more likely to occur where the tendon is attached to the bone in the heel.

Achilles tendinitis can develop even in people who are relatively inactive. It is not related to a specific injury, but a sudden increase in the intensity of an exercise or activity may trigger the condition. In both cases, the damaged fibers can harden. When the problem is at the heel, extra bone tissue (bone spurs) can develop.

Diagnosis and Treatment

As with most orthopaedic conditions, Achilles tendinitis is diagnosed by a combination of a physical examination, x-rays, and MRIs.

The evidence is not clear about the best ways to treat Achilles tendinitis, but the following suggestions are worth trying:

Give it a rest. Either cut back or stop doing what you think might have caused the Achilles tendon to become inflamed. If you really want to continuing exercising, find a low-impact substitute activity. A low impact exercise is one that does not put excess pressure on a joint. Riding a bike, using an elliptical machine, and swimming are examples.

Anti-inflammatory drugs like aspirin, ibuprofen, or naproxen might help with pain, as will ice applications for 20 to 30 minutes, several times a day. NSAIDs won't

Achilles Flex & Extend Stretch

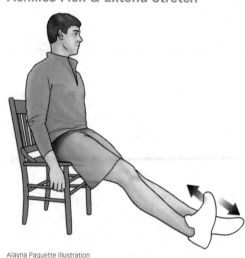

Alayna Paquette illustration

Stretch the Achilles tendon two to three times a day by flexing and extending the ankle. (See Chapter 5.)

reduce the thickening of tendon tissue, and they may have side effects that some people can't tolerate (bleeding and stomach distress) in the case of NSAIDs.

Easy exercises like the Achilles Wall Stretch (see illustration) may reduce pain and help avoid muscle spasms. Detailed instructions appear in Chapter 5. Exercise is safe if the heel is not swollen or tender, but be careful not to do too much, too soon. If it hurts, stop.

Here are some other treatment possibilities that your physician may recommend, although each has limitations:

Extracorporeal shockwave therapy (ESWT) involves high-energy impulses that stimulate the healing process, but the evidence of its effectiveness is not compelling.

Shoes and shoe inserts (orthotics) can balance the pressure being exerted on the affected area or provide additional support at the back of the shoe.

Cortisone injections are strong anti-inflammatory medications, but they are seldom used in the case of Achilles tendinitis.

Walking boots can help ensure that your tendon rests, but they should be used only for a short period of time.

Surgery is a last resort and is a seldom-used option.

Chronic Achilles tendinitis can result in an Achilles tendon rupture, discussed in the following section.

Achilles Tendon Rupture

A torn Achilles tendon occurs when there is a separation of the fibers so that the tendon can no longer function, according to the American Academy of Orthopaedic Surgeons. Under normal circumstances, the tendon can support 10 times a person's body weight.

You'll know when you suffer the injury. Patients report a snapping or popping sound at the back of the heel or the feeling of being kicked in the calf, accompanied by intense pain. You'll have difficulty walking and will suffer immediate loss of strength in the ankle.

The injury is most likely to occur in people ages 24 to 45, but it is not uncommon for an older, formerly sedentary person to tear the Achilles when he or she engages in a physically challenging activity.

Having had a prior ruptured Achilles tendon puts you in the high-risk category, as does previous treatment with corticosteroids in the area of the heel. Men sustain the injury five times more often than women.

Treatment

The immediate care for a torn Achilles tendon is ice, elevation, and over-the-counter pain medications. A medical professional should be sought.

If the tendon is completely torn (separated), you may need surgery, during which an incision is made and the torn tendon stitched together.

If it's a partial tear, according to the U.S. National Library of Medicine, your orthopaedic surgeon may recommend a cast, leg brace, splint, or boot for about six weeks. During that time, the tendon repairs itself by growing back together.

Rehab requires physical therapy, and most people return to their former level of activity within four to six months, according to the Mayo Clinic. Some problems persist as long as a year.

Achilles Wall Stretch

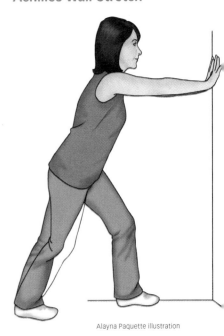

Alayna Paquette illustration

The Achilles wall stretch (see Chapter 5) can reduce stiffness and stress on the Achilles tendon.

Ruptured Achilles Tendon

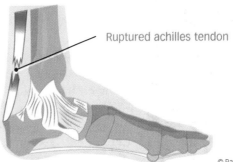

Ruptured achilles tendon

© Pawel Graczyk | Dreamstime

An Achilles tendon rupture may produce a snapping or popping sound. The American Orthopaedic Foot & Ankle Society notes that it can be repaired in outpatient surgery, but the patient can expect to wear a splint or cast from just below the knees down to the toes for around two weeks. If there are no complications, the patient may switch to a walking boot. A return to normal activities may take six months, a full recovery a year or more.

Prevention

Among the recommendations for preventing a torn Achilles are wearing correctly fitting shoes, shoes with a good arch support, and shoes that bend where your foot bends. The heel cushioning has to be just right—not so soft or low that your heel sinks lower than the front of your foot.

Stretch two or three times a day for 15 to 30 seconds at a time, as illustrated on the previous page and in Chapter 5. Stretch the lower legs before and after exercise. Start by simply walking slowly and gradually picking up the pace.

Bursitis (Heel)

Bursitis is an inflammation of the bursa—thin sacks of fluid that lubricate and cushion areas where structures rub against each other. It is most likely to affect the center of the heel. Older adults are more susceptible because bursae break down over time.

Causes

The condition can be caused by overuse, which in turn causes the bursae to become inflamed or irritated. Too much walking, jogging, or running are examples of overuse. Associated risks, according to the U.S. National Library of Medicine, are:

- Starting an intense workout.
- Suddenly increasing your activity level
- Changing your activity routine
- Having a history of arthritis

Symptoms

Symptoms include pain (especially when rising on the toes), warmth, and swelling that increases during the day. The pain may be worse when the ankle is bent upward.

Treatment

It begins with rest, ice, elevation, soft heels, supportive footwear, heel pads, prescription orthotics, and over-the-counter pain medications. The prognosis is good, but getting over bursitis may take several weeks of proper treatment.

Prevention

Stretch the Achilles tendon before and after exercise. Work on proper walking or jogging form. Use exercises in Chapter 5 to maintain strength and flexibility in the ankle joint, and wear shoes with enough arch support to minimize the inflammation in the bursae.

Claw Toe

Having a claw toe is as it sounds: Your toes claw, or dig into, the soles of your shoes, creating painful calluses.

Causes

Claw toes can be the result of nerve damage or from wearing shoes that squeeze your toes. Typical symptoms are:

- Toes bent upward from the joints at the ball of the foot
- Toes bent downward at the middle joints toward the sole of your shoe
- Toes bent downward at the top joints
- Corns that develop over the top of the toe or under the ball of the foot.

Treatment

- Wear shoes with soft, roomy toe boxes.
- Stretch your toes and toe joints toward their normal positions.
- Exercise your toes by using them to pick up marbles or a towel laid flat on the floor.

Special pads can redistribute your weight and relieve pressure. Try "in-depth" shoes that have an extra 3/8 of an inch in the toe box.

Dislocated Ankle

A dislocated ankle occurs when there is an abnormal separation between the three bones that constitute the ankle joint—the shinbone, the smaller bone in your lower leg, and the talus, which is a bone in the foot.

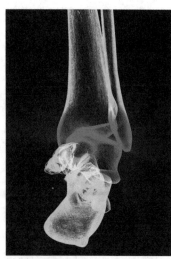

© jqbaker / Getty Images

Typically, a dislocated ankle involves fractures of the distal ends of the tibia and fibula bones, with collateral damage to the supporting ligaments.

Severe trauma can tear the ligaments that connect those bones and pull them out of place. They don't tear easily, and dislocations usually occur at the same time as a break, according to foot and ankle specialists at St. Luke's Hospital in Kansas City.

Symptoms

Symptoms, of course, won't be hard to notice. Here's the list:

- Immediate, severe pain
- Swelling
- Bruising
- Tenderness
- Difficulty moving the ankle
- Ankle deformity

Treatment

Treatment will include pain medications, elevation, and cold packs. If surgery isn't needed, a doctor will move the dislocated bones into place. In some cases, emergency surgery is needed, followed by use of a splint or cast to keep your ankle in place while it heals. Recovery takes six to 12 weeks.

Fallen Arches

The condition frequently called "fallen arches" is also known as adult-acquired flatfoot, according to the American Academy of Orthopaedic Surgeons (AAOS). It is one of the most common problems affecting the foot and ankle—one in five adults has it to some degree. Its symptoms are pain on the inside of the foot and ankle,

Achilles Flex & Extend Stretch

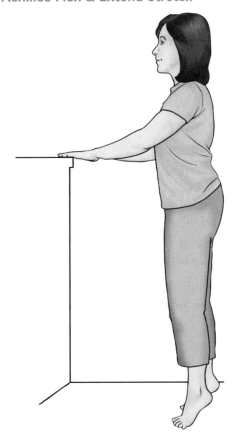

Alayna Paquette illustration

The toe-raise/calf-raise exercise (see Chapter 5) can relieve discomfort caused by fallen arches.

pain that is worse at night, and a heel bone that has shifted and puts pressure on the outside of the ankle bone. Other symptoms might be stiffness and a sensation of imbalance, especially if only one foot is affected.

See a doctor if you notice recently developed fallen arches. Pain may be relieved by supportive shoes, exercises (toe curls

Foot arch type

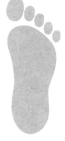
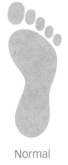
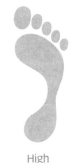

Flat   Normal   High   Very high

© Branchecarica | Dreamstime

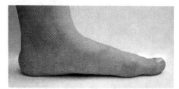

© игорь перекрестов | Dreamstime

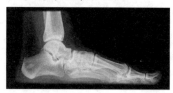

© Skyhawk911 | Dreamstime

While having flat feet won't necessarily cause problems, the condition may be a factor in such ailments as shin splints, tendinitis, and plantar fasciitis.

and heel raises), rest, ice after exercise, fitted insoles, shoes with low heels and wide soles, and orthotic inserts.

Don't ignore the problem. It could get worse and contribute to more pain—pain that can radiate up the legs and cause loss of balance.

Flat Feet

About 25 percent of Americans have flat feet, and most of them don't have a problem, according to the AAOS. However, people suffering from foot, knee, or leg pain, shin splints, Achilles tendinitis, or plantar fasciitis should pay attention to whether one foot is flatter than the other.

Flat feet vs. normal feet

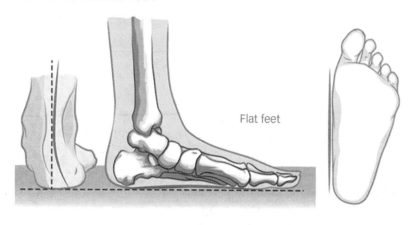

Flat feet

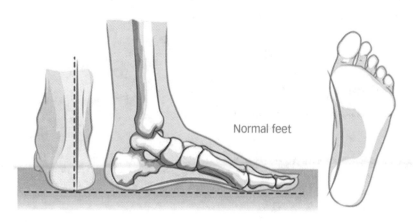

Normal feet

© Lukaves | Dreamstime

Having flat feet often is painless, but the condition can sometimes cause problems in the ankles and knees. Why? Because flat feet can alter the alignment of the legs. The tendons on the inside of the ankles—particularly the posterier tibial tendon (indicated by the vertical red line in illustrations at right)—have to work harder and are prone to extra pressure, which can cause painful, weak, or stiff feet and ankles.

Symptoms/Diagnosis

How do you know if you have flat feet? The simplest test is to check your wet footprint.

- If everything is normal, the front of your footprint should be joined to the heel by a strip about half the width of the front foot.
- If you have flat feet, that strip will be the same width as the front of your foot. Your footprint will look like a stretched-out pancake.
- If there's only a thin strip, that means you have a high arch.

You also can do a shoe evaluation to check for flat feet. Place your shoes on a flat table and examine them at eye level from behind, checking for even sole wear. A flat foot causes more wear on the inside of the sole, especially in the heel area. That type of wear causes the shoe to rock from side to side. And check the upper part of the shoes. A flat foot causes the upper part to lean inward toward the sole. If you suffer foot pain and have flat feet, see an orthopaedic surgeon or a podiatrist for an evaluation.

Treatment

Three things can be done about flat feet short of medical intervention:

- Wear shoes that have firm midsoles—the cushioning between the outer sole and the material that touches the foot.
- Wear shoes that have rigid heel counters—the stiff material at the back of the shoe.
- Wear shoes with good arch support. The worst choice for people with flat feet is highly cushioned shoes that do not provide stability.

In 95 percent of cases, orthotics (prescribed or customized shoe inserts) will reduce symptoms by at least 85 percent.

Being born with flat feet is not that unusual, but flat feet also can develop later in life. It's called adult-acquired flatfoot deformity. Surgery is a last-resort option to correct the condition, but it can be just as effective for older adults as for middle-aged and younger ones.

Hammertoes and Mallet Toes

The American Podiatric Medical Association (APMA) describes hammertoe as a bending of the toe at the first joint that makes the toe appear as an upside-down V when looked at from the side.

A mallet toe affects the joint nearest the toenail. Neither condition is likely to affect the big toe. The conditions are more common in women than in men.

Flexible hammertoes are less serious because they can be diagnosed and treated while still in the developmental stage. Rigid hammertoes are more developed and more serious. They are seen in people with severe arthritis and in those who waited too long to seek medical attention.

Causes

Hammertoes can be caused by tight footwear that crowds toes into a space that prevents them from lying flat. They also can be caused by trauma and by muscle imbalance that causes a toe to contract. Age, heredity, and length of toes also may be contributing factors.

Hammertoes might cause pain at the top of the bent toe, corns, swelling, redness, restricted motion, and pain in the ball of the foot.

NEW FINDING

Flatfoot Reconstruction Can Be Effective for Adults of Any Age

Physicians and scientists at the Hospital for Special Surgery presented findings that were the first to compare the outcomes of reconstruction for flat feet on older patients to those of a younger group. The study evaluated 130 patients over 65 with adult-acquired flatfoot deformity to determine if there were worse clinical outcomes or an increased number of subsequent surgical procedures when compared to younger patients. The younger groups included patients aged 45 to 65 (middle-aged) or less than 45 years old.

Overall, the findings did not demonstrate any differences in outcomes compared with patients in the middle-aged and younger groups. The authors believe a flatfoot reconstruction is a good option for patients regardless of age.

"Our initial hypothesis was that there would be increased complications for patients in the older group," said Scott J. Ellis, MD, senior study author. "However, we saw positive, consistent surgical outcomes across all age groups. Depending on the severity of the condition, we believe a flatfoot reconstruction is a great option for patients regardless of their age. For the right patient, it can be the last surgery that they need."

Presentation, American Academy of Orthopaedic Surgeons, March 2018

Treatment

The APMA suggests these home treatments:

- A non-medicated hammertoe pad
- Shoes with deep toe boxes
- Ice applications for pain and swelling
- Loose-fitting shoes

Medical treatment might involve padding and taping to minimize pain and address the muscle imbalance, anti-inflammatory drugs, cortisone injections, and custom shoe inserts. Surgical options are available to remove a bony prominence or restore normal alignment.

High Arches

Cavus foot is the medical term for a foot with an abnormally high arch. It places an excessive amount of weight on the

Hammertoes and mallet toes

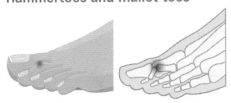

Hammertoes

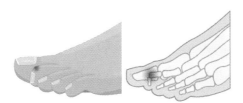

Mallet toes

© Aksana Kulchytskaya | Dreamstime

Hammertoes and mallet toes can result from tight footwear, trauma, muscle imbalance, age, and heredity.

High Arches

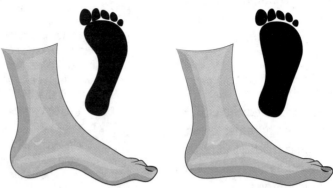

© Viktoria Kabanova | Dreamstime

High arches put too much pressure on the ball and heel, causing an unstable foot.

ball and heel of the foot when standing, according to the American College of Foot and Ankle Surgeons.

High arches may be caused by an inherited structural abnormality, a neurologic disorder, or medical conditions such as stroke, cerebral palsy, polio, and muscular dystrophy. The symptoms are hammertoes (bent toes), claw toes (clenched like a fist), calluses, pain when standing or walking, and an unstable foot that tilts inward. An unstable foot can lead to sprained ankles.

A foot and ankle surgeon can diagnose high arches by reviewing a patient's family history, a physical exam, and x-rays. Diagnosis may require an evaluation by a neurologist.

Non-surgical treatment options include orthotics for stability and cushioning the foot, modified shoes with high tops to support the ankle, and shoes wider on the bottom for greater stability. A brace may help keep the foot and ankle stable. Surgery is recommended only when conservative measures fail. It is done to decrease pain, increase stability, and compensate for weakness in the foot.

Osteoarthritis (OA)

You are nine times less likely to develop OA in the ankles than you are in the knees or hips, but it happens. Foot/ankle osteoarthritis is present in 17 percent of people over the age of 50, according to a January 2018 study in *Therapeutic Advances in Musculoskeletal Disease*.

Although cartilage in the ankle joint is damaged (as it is in other joints affected by OA), it is not the primary source of pain, because cartilage does not contain nerves. The pain and stiffness are caused by friction between bones.

Most cases of ankle OA are caused by a previous ankle injury (sprain, fracture) or an underlying medical condition (rheumatoid arthritis, for example).

Symptoms
- Ankle pain (also pain in the lower leg and pain in the back or middle of the foot)
- Stiffness
- Swelling
- Crunching or popping noise

Treatment
Treatment falls into four categories: lifestyle changes, medical interventions, joint injections, and surgery.

Lifestyle Factors
The first two lifestyle changes are just common sense. First, don't try to work through the pain. Give the ankle a rest. If you're doing something that makes the pain worse, stop and look for an alternative activity. Walking instead of jogging comes to mind.

Second, ice and/or heat are temporary fixes, but they're worth the effort. Use ice for 20 minutes after exercising and heat to ease the discomfort at other times.

The biggest, most difficult, and perhaps most important change is one you've probably heard before: Lose weight. Just one pound of excess weight puts five extra pounds of pressure on the ankle.

You'll know when it's time to go to the doctor if the pain doesn't subside after three days, it's getting worse, it recurs several times within a month, and/or it interferes with daily activities.

Medical Intervention

After a physical exam and perhaps blood tests to rule out other conditions, your doctor might recommend shoe inserts to reduce the pressure on the ankle or to support the joint. He might also order physical therapy that includes specific exercises to increase ankle flexibility and strength. You can safely do the exercises illustrated in Chapter 5 at home to both treat and prevent (or delay) joint problems. Detailed instructions for these exercises are included.

Injections

If neither exercises nor lifestyle changes have been effective, injections of a steroid or hyaluronic acid might be next. Steroids reduce swelling, stiffness, and pain but carry side effects that might not be acceptable. Most of the research supporting injections for joint OA has been on the knees, not the ankles. Evidence regarding dosages, strength, and frequency of ankle injections is sketchy.

Surgery

Most ankle OA problems can be treated without surgery. For those serious enough to warrant surgery, options include ankle debridement, ankle arthrodiastasis, ankle fusion, and ankle arthroplasty are options.

Debridement is basically cleaning up the ankle joint, removing inflamed tissue, trimming bone spurs, smoothing out

Osteoarthritis (OA)

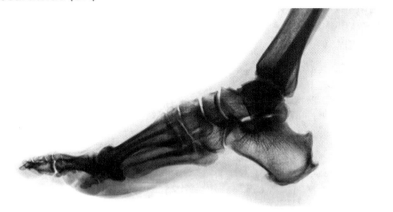

© Puwadol Jaturawutthichai | Dreamstime

Osteoarthritis is far more common in knees or hips, but it does affect the ankle as well, causing stiffness and pain in the joints, along with a crunching or popping noise.

remaining cartilage, and getting rid of loose bodies.

Arthrodiastasis is a procedure that implants an external fixation device for approximately 90 days to stretch the ankle joint and increase the space between bones in the foot and lower leg. It is then removed.

Fusion "welds" the tibia, fibula, and talus bones, eliminating bone friction and pain but reducing flexibility and possibly stressing other joints in the lower leg.

Ankle arthroplasty replaces, remodels, or adjusts the surface of the ankle joint, sometimes by trimming the problematic bone areas and/or adding different supportive materials.

Plantar Fasciitis (Heel Spur, Heel Pain)

Plantar fasciitis is an inflammation of the fibrous tissue (plantar fascia) that runs along the bottom of the foot. The longer the inflammation lasts, the more likely the lining of the heel also will be torn away.

The shelf-like structure that develops is as wide as the heel bone and is called a heel spur. The terms "plantar fasciitis" and "heel spurs" often are used interchangeably in common-day language.

Walkers, joggers, people with anatomical abnormalities, and those with tight calf muscles are in the high-risk group

Plantar Heel Pain: Manual Massage Therapy for Plantar Heel Pain

Is manual therapy consisting of deep massage, myofascial release, or joint immobilization effective for treating plantar heel pain (plantar fasciitis)? A review of studies, as reported in *The Foot*, set out to find the answer. Five of the studies showed a positive short-term effect after manual therapy treatment, mostly with a technique called soft tissue mobilization, with or without stretching exercises. Overall, the review determined that soft tissue mobilization is an effective method of treating plantar fasciitis.

The Foot, August 2017

for plantar fasciitis. Women are more likely to develop it than men, and being overweight is a risk factor for everyone.

Symptoms

The primary symptom of plantar fasciitis is heel pain. There also could be a feeling of a dull, dime-sized bruise buried in the heart of the heel. It usually hurts more in the morning and less during the day, and the pain intensifies with weight-bearing activity.

If a heel spur is present, you might feel a nodule at the point of pain. Some individuals also may report numbness, tingling, and swelling, but these symptoms are rare.

Causes

Although there are several theories about how it develops, plantar fasciitis is somewhat of a mystery. The ailment can seemingly materialize from nowhere.

Possible causes are excessive foot pronation (ankle rolling inward), shoes with worn-out heels, shoes that do not properly support the foot, running on hard or uphill surfaces, and dramatic increases in training intensity. It's often caused by the trauma to the heel that is associated with stepping on something like a rock.

Treatment

The healing process for plantar fasciitis can be agonizingly slow because the condition is aggravated with every step. Treatment includes rest, ice, anti-inflammatory pain medication, wearing cushioned pads under the heel, custom orthotics, and calf stretching exercises.

For the first few days, stretching can cause the pain to worsen, but eventually, flexibility exercises will lessen the pain. Manual massage, once considered an alternative treatment for plantar fasciitis, has become a more accepted mainstream or complementary approach.

Some physicians recommend wrapping the foot and ankle with an elastic bandage at a 90-degree angle before going to sleep at night. They also suggest immobilizing the foot at night with pillows. If the pain does not go away after six weeks, see a physician.

More aggressive treatment options are cortisone shots, walking casts, and extracorporeal shock wave therapy, but all three have either questions or limitations. If conservative treatment has failed after six months, you may want to consult an orthopaedic surgeon to discuss surgical options.

Plantar fasciotomy involves a procedure where a band of connective tissue is cut to relieve pressure on the troublesome area. However, the risks and benefits have to weighed by you in consultation with an orthopaedic surgeon to see if this route is appropriate.

Prevention

There is no conclusive evidence that stretches will prevent plantar fasciitis, but a systematic stretching program is generally a good idea for both the foot and the ankle.

You can continue exercising if you have plantar fasciitis, but only with activities that don't put pressure on the heel. Riding a stationary bicycle and swimming are two options.

Plantar Fasciitis

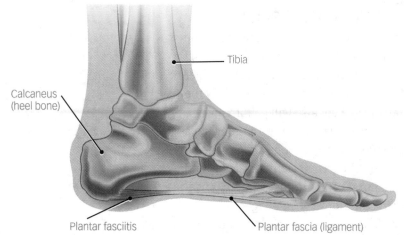

Tibia

Calcaneus (heel bone)

Plantar fasciitis

Plantar fascia (ligament)

© Rob3000 | Dreamstime

You'll know it if you've had it: the unmistakable heel pain of plantar fasciitis.

Rheumatoid Arthritis (RA)

More than 90 percent of rheumatoid arthritis patients develop symptoms in the foot and ankle over the course of their disease. Foot symptoms are the first sign of RA in 13 percent of patients.

The exact cause is unknown, but it is likely a combination of genetics and environmental factors that activate the disease. That's when the body's immune system attacks itself by producing substances that inflame the lining of the joints.

RA affects 1 percent of the population, occurring in women three times as often as in men. Symptoms usually begin to develop between the ages of 40 and 60.

Symptoms of Rheumatoid Arthritis

Any of the following symptoms can indicate RA in your ankle:

- Pain
- Swelling
- Stiffness
- Warmth in joints
- Corns, bunions
- Difficulty with inclines and stairs
- Symptoms that affect the same joints on each foot

Treatment

Prior to a recommending a treatment regimen, your doctor will do a conventional physical exam and look for skin issues, foot shape, tenderness to pressure, and joint flexibility.

Some people can control the symptoms with medications—aspirin, ibuprofen, methotrexate, prednisone, and sulfasalazine. Nonsurgical treatments include rest, ice, orthotics, braces, special shoes, exercise, and steroid injections.

Imaging is often required to further characterize the extent of joint degeneration and to see whether surgery is feasible or appropriate.

Surgical options for the ankle include fusion and, in advanced cases, total ankle replacement.

Fusion involves removing the joint and fusing two or more bones into one. Ankle replacement is for those who have had unsuccessful joint fusion surgery or where there is severe involvement of the joints in or near the ankle.

For the foot, the procedure depends on the location—hind-foot, mid-foot, or fore-foot—but it is still likely to involve fusion. The advantages of fusion are less pain and more stability. The disadvantage is less range of motion.

Sesamoiditis

Sesamoids are small, unique, pea-sized bones connected to other bones by tendons (instead of ligaments), or they are imbedded in muscles. Two of these sesamoids are in the bottom of the forefoot near the big (great) toe. They provide a smooth surface for tendons, assist in weight-bearing, and help elevate the bones of the big toe.

Sesamoids can be broken (fractured) or irritated and inflamed (sesamoiditis).

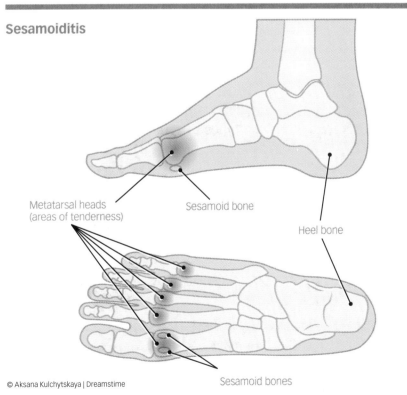

Sesamoiditis

Metatarsal heads (areas of tenderness)

Sesamoid bone

Heel bone

Sesamoid bones

© Aksana Kulchytskaya | Dreamstime

The sesamoid bones can be the source of inflammation that results in what's called sesamoiditis. The sesamoid bones also can be prone to fractures.

It is a form of tendinitis, according to the American Academy of Orthopaedic Surgeons, caused by repetitive movement, increased physical activity, and putting too much pressure on the balls of the feet.

Although sesamoiditis usually is associated with younger people and athletes, it also is seen in older adults with osteoarthritis and in people with high arches or "bony" feet. High arches add pressure; bony feet don't have enough fat to protect the sesamoids.

Symptoms

If a sesamoid bone is fractured, the pain is immediate. In sesamoiditis, the pain typically develops gradually or over a period of time. Other symptoms include possible bruising, difficulty in bending or straightening the big toe, swelling (but not always), and pain on the bottom of the foot.

Treatment

Treating sesamoiditis takes time (up to six weeks) but can almost always be done with at-home measures. It begins by stopping the activity that is causing the pain. Additional conservative treatments include:

- Over-the-counter pain medication (aspirin, ibuprofen)
- Ice applications 15 to 20 minutes at a time, two to three times a day
- Soft, low-heeled shoes
- Cushioned, in-shoe pads to relieve stress and pain
- Gradual return to normal activity

Your doctor may recommend taping the big toe so that it stays in a slightly downward position and/or a steroid injection to reduce inflammation and swelling.

Prevention

Wearing the right kinds of shoes is the best way to prevent sesamoiditis. Shoes should have a wide toe box and be comfortable, well-cushioned, and low-heeled. Padded socks may help. If you wear sneakers often, replace them often.

Sprained Ankle

The ankle is the most frequently injured part of the body among people who exercise. The severity of the injury ranges from one that allows you to return to normal activity in a few days to an injury that keeps you out of action for weeks at a time. Those who have had a sprained ankle are the ones most likely to suffer the same injury again.

A sprained ankle is a stretch tear or rupture of at least one of the ligaments

Types of sprained ankles

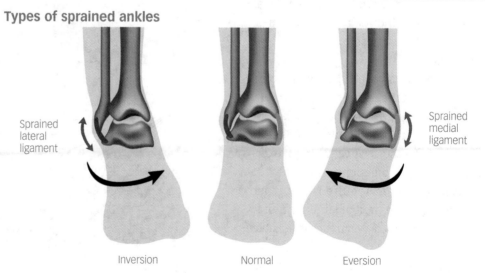

Sprained lateral ligament

Sprained medial ligament

Inversion   Normal   Eversion

© Alila07 | Dreamstime

Various types of sprains can affect different ligaments of the ankle.

that holds the bones of the ankle joint together. The tears might be microscopic or so large that they represent a complete disruption of the fibers.

One of the ligaments that wraps around the outside of the ankle is the weakest and the one most frequently injured. However, all three ligaments supporting the ankle, from front to back, can be sprained.

Symptoms of a Sprained Ankle

Sprained ankle symptoms vary according to the severity and grade of the sprain:

- **Grade 1 is minor strain with no tear.** It typically involves mild pain with some swelling.
- **Grade 2 is a partial tear.** It involves moderate pain, significant swelling, and some loss of motion)
- **Grade 3 is a full tear.** It's accompanied by severe pain and swelling and extreme loss of motion.

The best-case scenario is mild pain, localized swelling, and tenderness, but no instability. You can walk, but don't try to jump or jog. Grade 2 and 3 sprains involve not only greater pain, but sometimes a "popping" sound, bleeding, bruising, ankle instability, and difficulty walking.

Treatment of a Sprained Ankle

First-line of treatment for a sprained ankle is rest; ice (for 15 to 20 minutes at a time, three to four times a day); compression with an elastic bandage; wrap or support device; elevation; and pain medication.

Prevention of Sprained Ankles

Protective measures include wearing shoes with side-to-side support, bracing or taping the ankle, and following the 10 percent rule: Never increase an exercise's intensity or duration at a rate of more than 10 percent a week.

Sprained Foot

Harvard Medical School says foot sprains usually occur in two areas: the midfoot and the joint at the base of the big toe.

When it happens in the big toe, it's called turf toe (see the section titled Turf Toe). When it happens in the midfoot, it's simply called a sprain or midfoot sprain.

In mild or moderate cases of a sprained foot, there will be swelling, tenderness, and perhaps bruising. In severe sprains, you may not be able to stand or walk on the injured foot.

Treatment begins with rest, ice, compression, and elevation, plus NSAIDs (aspirin, ibuprofen, naproxen) for swelling and pain. More severe sprains may require immobilization. Return to normal activities gradually and with exercises to stretch and strengthen the muscles of the foot. Most sprains heal with time.

Strains

A muscle or tendon strain can occur in many areas of the body, including the foot or leg. A muscle or tendon can be stretched, partially torn, or completely torn. Activities that require a quick start put the lower leg, ankle, and foot at risk. Symptoms include pain, muscle spasms, muscle weakness, swelling, and inflammation.

The treatment is the same as for a sprain—rest, ice, compression, and elevation. With time and gradually progressive exercises, pain should subside and mobility will improve. Surgery is a consideration only in severe cases.

Stress Fractures

With so many bones in the foot and ankle, it is not surprising that they are the most common places to get stress fractures—small cracks in bones, frequently the metatarsals that connect the midfoot to the toes.

Among the people at higher risk are

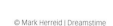

© Mark Herreid | Dreamstime

Above: A freshly sprained ankle needs ice—employ an ice pack for 15 to 20 minutes, three to four times per day. *Below*: Discoloring is a telltale sign of bad ankle sprains.

© Marc Bruxelle | Dreamstime

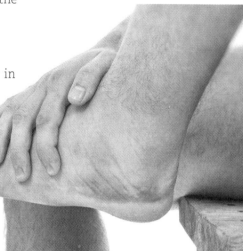

Sprained or Broken Toe?

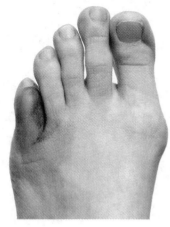

© Soupstock | Dreamstime

The symptoms are similar for both stubbed and broken toes.

sedentary individuals who suddenly begin a demanding exercise program, people who have diabetes or rheumatoid arthritis, and those who have osteoporosis or other conditions that result in weakened bones or decreased bone density.

People with healthy bones also can develop stress fractures in the foot if they repeat an activity over and over. A stress fracture is thought of as an overuse injury, but it could happen with nothing more than a change in physical activity. A physician may use x-rays or computerized tomography (CT) scans to make a diagnosis.

Symptoms of a stress fracture can include the following:

- A dull ache after exercise
- Swelling
- Pain that decreases only with rest and increases with activity
- Pain that gets progressively worse
- An area that is painful when pressure is applied

The first treatment is to stop the activity that caused the injury and avoid it for as long as six to eight weeks. Most stress fractures will heal with time and orthotic supports like shoe inserts or boot walkers.

Stubbed Toes and Broken Toes

Broken and stubbed (sprained) toes are common injuries usually caused by dropping a heavy weight on them or by leading with your toes when bumping into something. The symptoms are similar for both stubbed and broken toes.

Although very painful, stubbed toes don't always require a doctor visit. If you're not sure whether your toe is broken or stubbed, contact your doctor or go to a walk-in clinic. Typically, a technician will take an x-ray to see whether there is a fracture in the toe, and then your doctor will give you instructions based on the severity of the fracture. Typically, it will involve rest, ice, elevation, and OTC medications to relieve pain and limit swelling.

If it's just a stubbed toe (similar symptoms but not as severe or long-lasting), wear comfortable and loose shoes to prevent further damage.

If the toe fracture is nondisplaced, meaning the bone is cracked but is still in proper alignment, you can wrap the broken toe by placing soft padding between the toe and the one next to it ("the buddy toe") and taping them together. Don't wrap it too tightly.

If the big toe is broken (bleeding, bruising, numbness, tenderness, swelling, stiffness, decreased mobility), your doctor may want to put it in a cast for support. In some cases, surgery is needed for proper healing. Recovery takes four to six weeks.

Tendinitis

Tendinitis is inflammation of a tendon and, in the case of foot and ankle problems, the heel and ankle (see the "Achilles Tendinitis" section in this report). It is considered an "overuse" injury.

Tendinitis can happen to anyone,

The Foot Bones

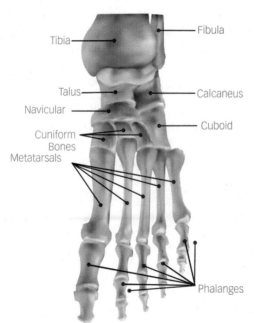

Tibia · Fibula · Talus · Calcaneus · Navicular · Cuboid · Cuniform Bones · Metatarsals · Phalanges

© Amphetamine500mg | Dreamstime

With so many bones, it's not surprising that the foot is such a common site of fractures.

but it's more common in adults who participate in sports. Older adults are susceptible because tendons lose elasticity and become weaker with age.

Symptoms

The symptoms are a dull ache, tenderness, and mild swelling. In addition to Achilles tendinitis, the condition can involve a tendon on the inner side of the ankle and inflammation of a tendon on the outer edge of the heel.

Treatment

Tendinitis usually responds to rest, physical therapy, ice and heat, and over-the-counter pain medications like aspirin, ibuprofen, and naproxen. Without treatment, tendinitis can develop into a rupture. If a tendon is ruptured, it may require surgery.

Prevention

Avoid walking on hard or uneven surfaces, choose low-impact exercises (bicycling, swimming), ice your ankle three times a day, 15 to 20 minutes at a time, and use cushioned heel inserts to absorb impact. Choose some of the exercises illustrated in Chapter 5 to stretch and strengthen the lower leg and ankles.

Turf Toe

Turf toe is a sprain of the connective tissue around the big toe. The sprain might damage ligaments or tendons, separately or in combination. It often occurs when the toe is bent and hyperextended when pushing off.

Turf toe often occurs on artificial surfaces; they're harder than grass and do not "give" as much when a force is placed on them. The injury is associated with football but can happen in any sport or activity.

Turf toe injuries can vary in severity from stretching of the soft tissue to partial tearing, and even total dislocation of the joint. Doctors grade the injuries like they

NEW FINDING

Misdiagnosed Foot and Ankle Injuries May Result in Arthritis, Chronic Pain, and Disability

A review of studies outlined subtleties that complicate identification and treatment of several conditions, including stress fractures and turf toe. The clinical signs of these conditions can be difficult to detect with standard imaging and can result in the improper treatment of foot and ankle trauma. These issues may lead to recurrent ankle sprains and tendinitis later on.

While many injuries can be treated with medications, immobilization, ice, and rest, others require surgery. Once a correct diagnosis is confirmed, the patient can be offered a range of options, from conservative to surgical.

Journal of the American Osteopathic Association, Jan. 30, 2017

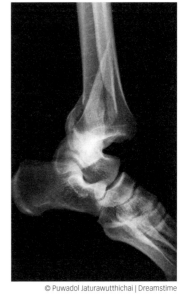

© Puwadol Jaturawutthichai | Dreamstime

A review of studies showed that incorrectly diagnosed foot and ankle conditions can result in recurrent complications.

grade other sprains—1 to 3, mild to severe (see sidebar on page 30).

Causes

Turf toe can occur in any sport or activity when the forefoot is fixed on the ground, the heel is raised, and a force pushes the big toe into a hyperextended position. The injury is traumatic—you'll know exactly when it happens.

Turf toe

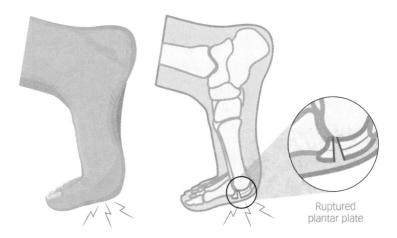

© Aksana Kulchytskaya | Dreamstime

Ruptured plantar plate

The hyperextension of the big toe when pushing off can result in turf toe, which can vary in severity from sprains to a rupture of the plantar plate of the big toe.

Grading the Severity of Turf Toe*

- **Grade 1:** The area surrounding the joint, called the plantar complex, has been stretched and causes tenderness and slight swelling.

- **Grade 2:** A partial tear of the plantar complex causes widespread tenderness, swelling, and bruising. Movement of the toe is limited and painful.

- **Grade 3:** The plantar complex is completely torn, causing severe tenderness, swelling, and bruising. Trying to move the big toe is difficult and painful.

*Adapted from the American Academy of Orthopaedic Surgeons

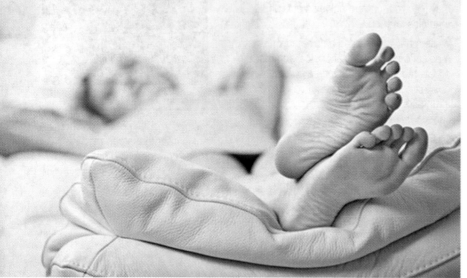

© Mark Herreid | Dreamstime

Elevation, a key component of the RICE protocol (see below), is critical for treatment of turf toe and other foot and ankle injuries.

Treatment

The RICE protocol is effective for Grade 1 turf toe. It bears repeating, letter by letter:

- **Rest**—Take a break from the activity that caused the injury and avoid walking or putting weight on your foot.

- **Ice**—Use cold packs for 20 minutes at a time, several times a day.

- **Compression**—Wear an elastic compression bandage to help prevent additional swelling.

- **Elevation**—Recline when you rest, and put your leg up higher than your heart.

In addition, over-the-counter anti-inflammatory medications such as ibuprofen can help provide relief from symptoms.

Grade 2 sprains may require immobilization. You may need a walking boot for at least the first week. After that, the injury is treated with taping.

Grade 3 injuries require immobilization for several weeks with a walking boot or cast that keeps the big toe pointing in a partially down position.

Recovery time ranges from a few weeks to a few months.

Surgery is rarely performed for turf toe but may be an option when other measures don't resolve the problem. Surgery could address a severe tear, a fracture, instability, loose bone chips, cartilage damage, and a new or worsening bunion.

Prognosis

When turf toe is treated early, the injury typically heals well. Joint pain and joint stiffness are the most common complications.

What's Next?

Chapter 3 describes 17 non-orthopaedic conditions—how they're identified, treated, and, in some cases, prevented.

A Closer Look: 6 Common Causes of Ankle Pain

We've all heard about the Achilles heel. That code word for vulnerability can also be applied to the ankle, an intricate system of bones and joints that is the linchpin of mobility and independence.

By Helen Boehm Johnson, MD, for University Health News

Our ankles are complex structures composed of four bones—the tibia and fibula (bones of the lower leg), the calcaneus (heel bone), and the talus (a small bone between the tibia, fibula, and calcaneus), along with multiple tendons and ligaments. Cushioning between the ankle's bones is provided by articular cartilage, which covers the ends of the bone where they intersect, and synovium, a thin tissue that lines the spaces between the bones and that secretes a lubricating fluid (synovial fluid). Damage to any of these components, whether from injury or disease, results in ankle pain. Common causes:

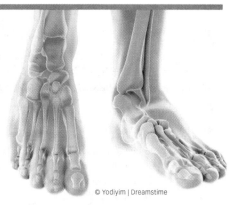

© Yodiyim | Dreamstime

People who have had severe ankle sprains in the past may suffer from instability and are prone to future sprains.

1 Sprains. A sprain occurs when a ligament is stretched beyond its normal range, causing injury to the ligamentous tissue. The most common ligaments involved in ankle sprains are the anterior talofibular ligament and calcaneal fibular ligament on the lateral or outside aspect of the ankle. Approximately half of all ankle sprains occur in athletes and usually involve twisting, rolling, or turning of the foot.

When the ligament is severely stretched, the ligamentous fibers can actually tear. A partial tear of the ligament is called a grade 2 sprain; a complete tear is called a grade 3 sprain. A grade 1 sprain results from a ligament that has been excessively stretched but not torn.

Pain, swelling, bruising, and tenderness are common ankle sprain symptoms. Most sprains are diagnosed by physical exam and treated with rest, compression dressings, and pain-relief medications such as non-steroidal anti-inflammatory drugs (NSAIDs). Some grade 3 sprains may require surgical repair of the ligament.

2 Fractures. Ankle fractures can involve any or all of the bones that make up the ankle joint: the tibia, fibula, and talus. Fractures can occur by many of the same mechanisms that cause sprains: abnormal twisting, rolling, or turning of the ankle or foot.

Symptoms of ankle fracture can mimic those of sprains, which is why most experts recommend that any ankle injury be evaluated by a doctor. X-rays are most often used to diagnose ankle fracture. Depending on the severity of the fracture, the bones involved, and the stability of the joint, treatment may range from rest to

immobilization of the joint to surgery using metal screws, rods, or wiring.

3 Gout. Gout is a disease in which uric acid crystals accumulate in different joints of the body, causing intense pain. It most commonly affects the joint of the big toe, a condition called podagra, but it can affect the ankle joint as well, causing severe pain. The pain is often sudden in onset (hence the phrase "gout attack," a condition that in some can be averted via diet changes), and the ankle may become warm and swollen. In people with chronic gout, uric acid crystals may accumulate under the skin, forming hard, lumpy protrusions around the ankle.

Gout treatment can involve pain control with NSAIDs, inflammation reduction with steroids, and a medication called colchicine. A "gout diet" (one low in purine-rich foods) can help prevent future attacks.

4 Rheumatoid Arthritis. Rheumatoid arthritis (RA) is an autoimmune disease in which the body's immune system attacks the synovial lining of joints, causing pain, swelling, stiffness, and, in some cases, joint deformity. More than 90 percent of people suffering from RA will have involvement of the foot or ankle at some point, and typically, both feet or both ankles are affected. When the ankle is involved, people will initially have difficulty with inclines (e.g., climbing stairs). Ultimately, the act of just walking or standing can cause significant ankle pain.

Your physician likely will treat the underlying disease with NSAIDs, cyclooxygenase 2 inhibitors (COX-2 inhibitors), steroids, and/or disease-modifying anti-rheumatic drugs (DMARDs) and by using special

orthotics and braces to stabilize the ankle. If RA results in significant deformity of the ankle joint, surgical repair of stretched or distorted tendons may be necessary.

5 Osteoarthritis. Even though osteoarthritis is the most common form of arthritis, it's a rare cause of ankle pain. When it does occur, destruction of cartilage between the bones of the ankle can cause pain and stiffness. Ankle osteoarthritis is treated with NSAIDs or COX-2 inhibitors, among other pain relief medications. Rarely, steroid injections into the ankle joint are used to control pain and reduce inflammation.

6 Psoriatic Arthritis. Psoriatic arthritis is an autoimmune form of arthritis that can occur in individuals suffering from the skin condition psoriasis, which is characterized by silvery, scaly skin lesions. Any joint in the body—and particularly the ankle—can be affected. The result: pain, stiffness, and swelling of the ankle. Treatment is similar to that for rheumatoid arthritis and includes treating the underlying disease with DMARDs, pain control with NSAIDs, and supportive care of the ankle with orthotics or braces.

Plus...
Less common causes of ankle pain include pseudogout (caused by calcium pyrophosphate dehydrate crystals in the ankle joint), lupus, infectious arthritis (a.k.a. septic arthritis), and reactive arthritis (an arthritis that follows an infection of the gastrointestinal, urinary, or genital system).

Helen Boehm Johnson is a medical writer who brings the combined experience of a residency-trained physician and an undergraduate English major to her work.

A Closer Look: 8 Common Causes of Heel Pain

Seven percent of Americans over 65 experience heel pain. Causes range from localized injuries to consequences of systemic disease.

By Helen Johnson, MD, for University Health News

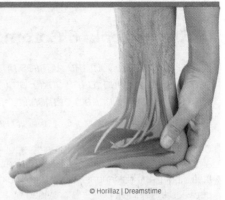

© Horillaz | Dreamstime

People tend to think of the heel—sometimes called the "hindfoot"—first as a bone (it's also called the calcaneus). But there are many different types of tissue that make up the heel. Disorders of any of these tissues and the structures they form can be a source of heel pain. From localized injuries to consequences of systemic disease, a variety of reasons can cause heel pain:

1 **Plantar Fasciitis.** The plantar fascia is a fibrous piece of tissue connecting the heel bone to bones of the toes. It plays a critical role in the biomechanics of foot strike and foot push-off. Irritation and injury of the plantar fascia are the most common causes of heel pain.

Causes of plantar fasciitis include overuse through activities like running, prolonged standing, arch abnormalities (too high or too low), prolonged wearing of shoes with insufficient arch support, obesity, fibromyalgia, and inflammatory arthritides. As those who have experienced the condition can attest, the pain of plantar fasciitis is usually worse in the morning, when you're taking your first few steps out of bed, but it improves over the course of the day.

Treatment involves icing, non-steroidal anti-inflammatory drugs (NSAIDs), and rest initially, followed by stretching and walking as symptoms improve. Some 90 percent of people with plantar fasciitis will improve within two months of starting treatment. Some cases may require a steroid injection, a foot boot to keep the foot flexed during sleep, or even surgery.

2 **Achilles Tendonitis.** The Achilles tendon is formed by fibers of the calf muscles that insert onto the back of the calcaneus. Inflammation of this tendon often occurs after overuse of the calf muscles, particularly in athletes who run and jump frequently. Patients with Achilles tendonitis often have tenderness and swelling at the back of the heel, where the tendon inserts. It's usually accompanied by pain when flexing the foot upward (dorsiflexion). Treatment involves NSAIDs, the use of orthotics, and physical therapy.

3 **Bursitis.** There are two bursae in the heel: the retrocalcaneal bursa, which lies between the calcaneus and the Achilles tendon, and the retroachilles bursa, which lies between the Achilles tendon and the skin. Both can become inflamed and cause heel pain.

The most common cause of inflammation of these bursae comes from ill-fitting shoes with a stiff edge that irritates the bursae. Less common causes of heel bursitis are rheumatoid arthritis (RA)—a disease in which the immune system attacks and damages the synovial lining of joints—and Achilles tendonitis. Treatment depends on the etiology, or set of causes, of the bursitis. A change in footwear could be to blame, as could NSAIDs you're taking for bursitis caused by shoes.

4 **Nerve Disorders.** Diseases such as diabetes, which can cause peripheral neuropathy, may result in heel pain. The most common cause of nerve-related heel pain, however, is tarsal tunnel syndrome, a condition whereby the posterior tibial nerve travels down the leg, dividing into several branches as it passes through the ankle region.

The space in the ankle region through which these branches pass is called the tarsal tunnel, and it's formed by the calcaneus, another bone of the foot called the talus, and a fibrous band of tissue. Damage to the branches of these nerves—often caused by compression and entrapment in this tunnel or from stretching of the nerves from collapse of the foot arch (flatfoot)—can cause heel numbness, pain, or tingling.

Treatment for nerve-related heel pain involves resting your affected foot, taking NSAIDs, and doing stretching exercises. Surgical decompression of the nerve may be necessary in rare cases.

5 **Heel Pad Disorders.** The heel pad, a shock-absorbing structure under the calcaneus, is composed of fat and fibrous tissue. A so-called "stone bruise" can occur when you step or land forcefully on a hard object, resulting in a painful bruise of the heel pad. Excessive pressure on the pad from obesity also can result in pain and soreness of the heel. The most often-prescribed treatments include rest and pain control with NSAIDs.

6 **Stress Fractures.** Stress fractures of the calcaneus can cause heel pain and are most common in participants of sports that involve frequent running or jumping. Stress fractures also can occur in people with low bone density (osteopenia or osteoporosis) who are at increased risk for fractures in general. Treatment involves rest and, for some, non-weight-bearing assistance devices such as crutches, along with NSAIDs or other analgesics for pain control.

7 **Infection.** Osteomyelitis—an infection of bone— can occur in the calcaneus and is a rare cause of heel pain. It is more common in people with diabetes or peripheral vascular disease. Patients may have an open sore or wound on the foot in addition to redness, swelling, and occasionally systemic symptoms of infection such as fever. Treatment involves antibiotics.

8 **Systemic Diseases.** A variety of different systemic diseases can be sources of heel pain. Among them: rheumatoid arthritis and gout. Osteoarthritis, the most common form of arthritis, rarely causes heel pain; it's more likely to cause toe or midfoot pain.

Helen Boehm Johnson is a medical writer who brings the combined experience of a residency-trained physician and an undergraduate English major to her work.

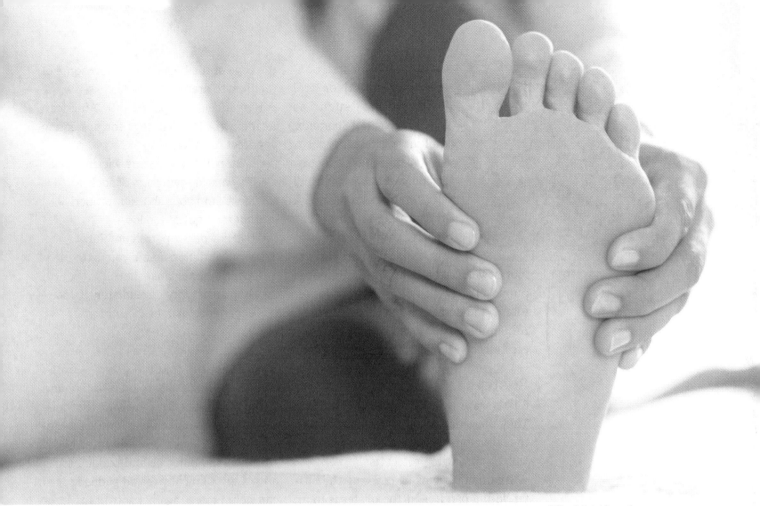

© Siam Pukkato | Dreamstime

Do you pay enough attention to your feet? Beyond the orthopaedic conditions discussed in Chapter 2, there are all kinds of issues we can affect with proper foot care; 17 of them are highlighted in this chapter.

3 Non-Orthopaedic Foot and Ankle Conditions

The 17 conditions listed alphabetically in this chapter are non-orthopaedic in nature. They can affect bones, muscles, and the structures surrounding joints and can cause just as much discomfort as orthopaedic issues.

Athlete's Foot

Athlete's foot is more common in men than in women and more common in older adults than in other age groups. It is a fungal infection that affects up to 15 percent of the population. Bacterial and fungal infections develop because feet spend a lot of time in the perfect breeding ground of warm, dark, humid shoes.

You'll recognize the symptoms of athlete's foot. They include redness, small blisters, itching, burning, and/or peeling. Once these infections develop,

they are hard to cure. Over-the-counter medications include such products as Desenex, Lamisil AT, Lotrimin Ultra, and Tinactin.

If things don't get better within two weeks, see your doctor. He or she might

Non-Orthopaedic Foot & Ankle Conditions

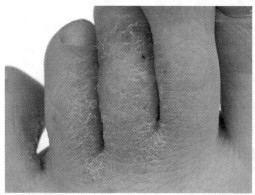

© Carroteater | Dreamstime

The redness, itching, and burning of athlete's foot should clear up with over-the-counter remedies within a couple of weeks.

The swelling and inflammation of bunions can become annoying and painful. The condition can end up requiring medical care in the form of drugs or even cortisone shots.

© Vienybe | Dreamstime

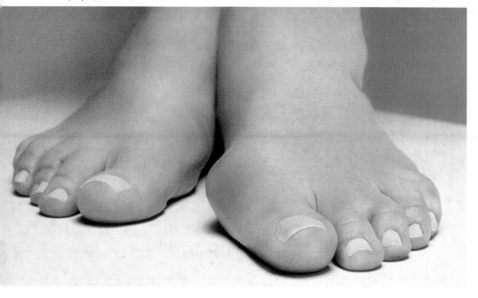

recommend prescription-strength topical or oral medications such as Lamisil, Micatin, Sporanox, Naftin, or Diflucan.

Prevent athlete's foot by keeping your feet clean and dry. Wear socks that wick moisture away from the feet. Change shoes, socks, or stockings often and use foot powder daily. Don't walk barefoot in public places. Wear flip-flops in locker rooms and showers. One other warning: Athlete's foot that has been treated successfully can come back.

Blisters

Blisters are usually caused by friction. They are small pockets filled with fluid that develop on the upper layer of skin, which is trying to protect itself.

Treatment begins by covering the blister with a bandage. If the blister is in an area of the foot that can be protected, use padding to protect it. Cut the padding into a donut shape with a hole in the middle, then place it around the blister. Cover the padding with a bandage. Avoid popping or draining a blister, if possible. It could lead to infection.

If a blister is large and painful, sterilize a small needle with rubbing alcohol, pierce the edge of the blister, and allow some of the fluid to drain.

Here are some tips from the American Academy of Dermatology for protecting your feet from blisters:

- Wear nylon or moisture-wicking socks.
- Try wearing two pairs of socks.
- Make sure your shoes fit properly—not too tight or too loose.
- Use powder or petroleum jelly to reduce friction where your skin rubs together or against shoes.
- Stop an activity immediately if you experience pain or discomfort or your skin turns red.

Bruises

It's almost impossible to prevent foot and ankle bruises, but there are ways to reduce the risk, according to the Institute for Preventive Foot Health. Properly fitted shoes with non-slip outsoles and padded socks are a start. Clinically-tested padded socks can help protect against soft tissue injuries because they diminish the effects of impact and pressure forces.

The symptoms are familiar—tenderness to touch, swelling, and color that changes from blue to purple to yellowish.

Most (light) bruises heal on their own. Ice and elevation may reduce or prevent swelling. If you suspect a deeper bone bruise, contact your doctor.

Bunions

Bunions develop when the joints of the big toe become deviated outwards and often become swollen and tender. If a bunion is not severe, wearing widely cut shoes or pads to cushion the bunion might work. Avoiding activities that require being on your feet for long periods of time reduces the risk. Ice can provide relief from inflammation and pain.

Shoe inserts are another alternative. Doctors might recommend over-the-counter drugs, prescribe anti-inflammatory drugs, or give cortisone shots to relieve the pain.

Less frequently, same-day surgery can relieve pressure and repair the joint in more severe cases. During surgery, bones, ligaments, tendons, and nerves are put back along correct direction, and the bump is removed.

Corns and Calluses

Corns and calluses affect about 5 percent of people in the U.S. Both conditions involve a thick outer layer of skin, and both can be caused by pressure or toes rubbing together. They also may result from foot deformities caused by rheumatoid arthritis or misshapen toes.

The difference is that corns (and there are five types of them) have a core and normally develop on a knobby part of a toe, while calluses are evenly distributed on the soles of the feet. Although some calluses may protect a part of the foot, both corns and calluses can be big enough to cause pain and difficulty in walking.

When they are painful, the goal in treating corns is to reduce or eliminate the pressure or friction that causes them. Wear shoes that fit, use pads that cushion the area, and use an over-the-counter product that contains salicylic acid. It softens the tissue, making it possible to remove the dead skin. Curad, Mediplast, and Dr. Scholl's Corn and Callus Remover are trade names.

If you have diabetes, peripheral artery disease, or peripheral neuropathy, get medical attention for corns or calluses.

Diabetes

Diabetes can contribute to other problems, including osteoporosis and neuropathic arthropathy.

Neuropathic arthropathy is a complication of diabetes in which a joint deteriorates because of nerve damage. The condition primarily affects the feet. It is treated by controlling blood sugar levels and physical therapy.

People with type 1 diabetes are at an increased risk of osteoporosis. Osteoporosis causes a lack of bone density that makes victims prone to fractures. The feet and ankles are the most common sites of a stress fracture, according to the Hospital for Special Surgery.

Stress fractures due to osteoporosis rarely involve major trauma. It's usually from normal activity and minor trauma. Treatment does not usually require surgery, but you might have to wear a boot or brace until the fracture heals.

The growing number of diabetics, combined with the epidemic of obesity, is increasing the incidence of Charcot foot, a condition that typically occurs in diabetics who have nerve damage. A study conducted at Loyola Medicine in Chicago found that nearly four out of five diabetic patients with severe cases of Charcot foot were able to walk normally following surgery.

A separate study published in *Clinical Diabetes and Endocrinology* (February 2017) found that 67 percent of endocrinologists, internal medicine physicians, and family medicine physicians described themselves as having poor or complete lack of knowledge of Charcot foot.

Gout

More than 8 million Americans suffer from bouts of gout. When an episode of gout develops, it can cause excruciating pain—usually in the big toe—but the discomfort subsides with or without treatment in five to 15 days.

Although the pain goes away, the attacks come back within a year in most people. Others may not experience a flare for years.

Causes

The condition is caused by excessive amounts of uric acid and the needle-like crystal deposits that are left behind. The increase in uric acid can happen because too much is being produced and the kidneys cannot efficiently remove it from the body.

NEW FINDING

High Success Rate for Diabetic Charcot Foot Surgery

Approximately 80 percent of diabetic patients with charcot foot were able to walk normally following surgery, according to researchers at Loyola Medicine in Chicago. Charcot foot typically occurs in diabetics who have nerve damage. Also called diabetic foot, charcot foot can develop following a minor injury such as a sprain or stress fracture and can result in severe deformities or bone infections. Among 214 patients who underwent surgery over a 12-year period, 173 of 223 feet had good or excellent outcomes. A common treatment for the condition is to put the patient in a cast, but bones can heal in deformed positions or collapse under the patient's weight. The surgical technique developed at Loyola may allow patients to avoid that risk.

Foot & Ankle International, March 27, 2018

Gout

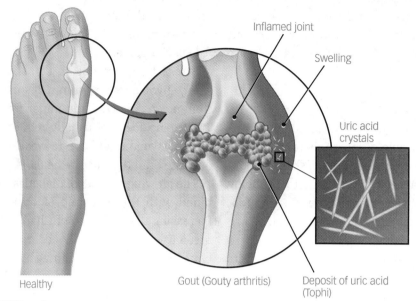

Inflamed joint

Swelling

Uric acid crystals

Healthy

Gout (Gouty arthritis)

Deposit of uric acid (Tophi)

© Rob3000 | Dreamstime

Gout—often striking in the joint of the big toe—affects men more often than women. The first bout can hit between the ages of 30 and 50.

Risk Factors

- Alcohol consumption
- Gender (men more likely than women)
- Age (30 to 50 for the first bout)
- Being overweight (BMI over 25)
- Race (African-American men twice as likely to report gout than Caucasian men)

Primary gout is the most common form, and those that have it usually have a family history of gout. It develops between the ages of 30 and 60. Secondary gout occurs as a result of long-term treatment with diuretics. It is usually found in patients 65 and older and is often associated with osteoarthritis.

Certain types of foods, beverages, and medications can't directly cause gout, but they can raise the level of uric acid. These include shellfish, red meats, refined carbohydrates such as white bread, processed foods such as chips, alcohol in excess, drinks and foods high in sugar content, and medications such as low-dose aspirin, certain diuretics (Esidrix), and immunosuppressants used in organ transplants such as cyclosporine (Neoral, Sandimmune).

Treatment

Two recent studies show that diet and medications could delay, minimize, or even prevent an attack.

One study found that the DASH diet (Dietary Approaches to Stop Hypertension) is associated with a lower risk of gout than a typical Western diet.

The other study, published by the American Academy of Family Physicians,

NEW FINDING

DASH Diet May Reduce the Risk of Gout

A study led by Massachusetts General Hospital investigators found that the DASH diet (Dietary Approaches to Stop Hypertension) is associated with a lower risk of gout. Food frequency questionnaires of more than 44,000 men were used to classify those who followed a DASH diet and those who chose a predominantly Western diet. (A DASH diet is high in vegetables, nuts, legumes, low-fat dairy products, and whole grains. The Western diet is based on a high intake of red and processed meats, French fries, refined grains, sweets, and desserts.) Men in both groups were monitored for 26 years to determine the incidence of gout. The DASH diet was associated with a significantly lower risk, suggesting that its effect of lowering uric acid levels translated into a lower risk of gout. The Western diet was linked with a higher risk of gout. Changing it may be a preventive approach for those at risk.

BMJ, May 9, 2017

How to Treat Gout in Your Foot

If you've ever woken up with severe pain in the base of your big toe, instep, or ankle, you may have had gout—and could be at risk of future flares.

By Leonaura Rhodes, MD, for University Health News

Gout in foot, instep, and ankle areas is common, affecting up to 8 million Americans today. The condition has been recorded throughout history, affecting many famous people—the most notorious of whom was Henry VIII, renowned for his lavish diet of rich food and copious amounts of alcohol.

What Is Gout?

It's an inflammatory arthritis—some call it "gouty arthritis"—caused by the formation of needle-like uric acid crystals in the joint.

Hyperuricemia (high blood urate levels) leads to crystal formation and severe episodes of acute pain, stiffness, tenderness, warmth, redness, and swelling, often striking along the base of the big toe.

The Pathology of Gout

Gout is primarily a metabolic disorder in which uric acid (also known as urate) accumulates in blood (hyperuricemia) and tissues.

When tissue levels reach saturation, crystals form, causing inflammation. This occurs most commonly in the cooler joints, notably the metatarsophalangeal joint of the big toe.

Many people with hyperuricemia never develop gout, but those with the highest levels are most likely to suffer episodes.

Symptoms and Signs of Gout

An attack of gout is often sudden and accompanied by telltale symptoms. It may present with excruciatingly painful swelling of joints (in the big toe, it is known as podagra). The joint may be stiff and appear red or purple, very swollen, and tender to even light touch.

An attack often begins at night; the acute phase lasts up to 12 hours. If untreated, the inflammation may last up to two weeks. Kidney stones precede the onset of gout in 14 percent of patients. And skin may peel and itch as healing begins.

Some people have a single attack of gout, while others are affected intermittently, often when they have overindulged or experienced dehydration. Chronic gout may develop, and it may affect more than one joint, mimicking rheumatoid arthritis. In its chronic form, gout can cause irreversible damage to the joints, tendons, and other soft tissue.

Treatment of Gout

Your doctor will determine your gout treatment, perhaps using American College of Rheumatology (ACR) guidelines:

Initial treatment. In an acute attack, a combination of NSAIDs (nonsteroidal anti-inflammatory drugs), corticosteroids, and

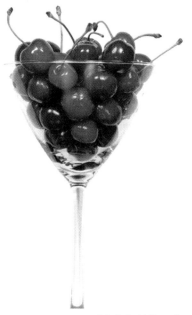

© Emilia Stasiak | Dreamstime

You can ease gout symptoms with a healthy diet—one that includes such choices as cherries and vitamin C foods and that limits such choices as legumes, red meat, and seafood (see "Gout Diet" list below).

colchicine may be needed. Steroids can be given orally or injected into the muscle or joint. Rest, elevation, ice packs, and increasing water intake may help.

Colchicine is a drug that decreases swelling and reduces the buildup of uric acid crystals. Side effects are common and include nausea, vomiting, and diarrhea.

Urate-lowering-treatment (ULT) is usually commenced after an attack. These drugs may be considered if colchicine is not effective, if multiple joints are involved, or if there is a history of kidney stones. ULT drugs include allopurinol (Aloprim), febuxostat (Uloric), and probenecid (Benemid).

Lifestyle change. Many people with gout benefit from lifestyle change. Regular exercise and eating a healthy diet not only will help you reach a healthy weight but also may reduce gout flare-ups.

Leonaura Rhodes, MB ChB, MPH, is a physician-turned-author who serves as Belvoir Media Group's medical editor. She's a frequent contributor to University Health News and Belvoir's health report division.

Gout Diet: What Helps, and What to Avoid

INCREASE:

- Water intake (good hydration may prevent attacks)
- Vitamin C in food or as a supplement
- Coffee (regular caffeinated coffee, in moderation)
- Cherries (which can lower the risk of recurrence by up to 35 percent)
- Fresh vegetables, salads, and fruits (excluding those on the "Restrict" list).

RESTRICT:

- Red meat and organ meats (offal)
- Seafood, especially anchovies, herring, sardines, mussels, scallops, trout haddock, mackerel, and tuna
- Yeast and yeast extracts
- Legumes (beans, peas, lentils)
- Spinach, asparagus, cauliflower, and mushrooms
- Alcohol, especially beer
- Processed foods, particularly those containing high fructose corn syrup.

Febuxostat Reduces the Risk of Gout Flares

The drug febuxostat reduced gout flares in a study of 314 adults with early gout, according to a study conducted at the University of Auckland. Febuxostat controls high urate levels in the blood. Febuxostat treatment also reduced inflammation of the joint lining detected by MRI scanning over a two-year period when it was compared to treatment with a placebo. Current clinical guidelines do not recommend routine use of urate-lowering therapy for people after the first gout flare. Dr. Nicola Dalbeth, lead author of the study, says this study indicates that even for people who have had one or two prior gout flares, urate-lowering therapy to reduce serum urate below 6 milligrams per deciliter may be beneficial in reducing future flares, Dr. Dalbeth said.

Arthritis & Rheumatology, Oct. 4, 2017

concludes that using medications to manage gout as a chronic condition (rather than as individual episodes) could help prevent recurrences.

Two medications that prevent the production of uric acid are allopurinol (Zyloprim) and febuxostat (Uloric). In 2017, the FDA approved a combination of allopurinol and lesinurad (Zurampic) for gout-associated high levels of uric acid.

Physicians can be more proactive in treating their patients' gout as a chronic condition requiring frequent monitoring than treating it as a series of isolated but inevitable episodes. Patients have to make the decision themselves, however, to more closely follow DASH diet guidelines.

Ingrown Toenail

Ingrown toenails are potentially painful but surprisingly treatable, according to the American College of Foot and Ankle Orthopedics & Medicine (ACFAOM). They develop when the skin on the side of a toenail grows over the edge of the nail or when the nail curls and grows into the skin. The toenail on the big toe seems to be the most vulnerable.

The most common cause is cutting toenails so that they grow at an angle into the skin instead of trimming them straight across. The nail eventually punctures the skin and causes pain and other symptoms. Other factors that can lead to the problem are nails that are too large for the toe, toes that curl, and trauma to the toe.

Symptoms

Ingrown toenail symptoms develop gradually and begin with minor pain and tenderness. But the condition progresses to the point where wearing certain shoes becomes uncomfortable or intolerable. Swelling, a discharge, and a feeling that is hot to the touch can mean that the area has become infected. The sooner you recognize the symptoms, the better your chances to resolve the problem with at-home treatment.

Treatment

If you have diabetes, see your primary care doctor or podiatrist right away, no matter how minor the problem. For everyone else, the ACFAOM recommends the following treatment:

- Clean the foot with soap and water.
- Apply a mild antiseptic.
- Bandage the toe, but not too tightly.
- Repeat the procedure three times a day.
- Use over-the-counter medications to harden the skin and shrink the soft tissue along the edge of the nail.
- Use special commercial bandages to cushion the area.

If that doesn't work, contact a podiatric physician or surgeon. He or she can trim or remove an infected nail, or reshape the nail to make it narrower and less likely to grow into the skin.

Prevention

To prevent ingrown toenail issues, follow these practices:

- Trim your toenails straight across.
- Don't cut the sides of toenails.
- Never pick or pull at a toenail.
- Wear shoes with adequate room in the toe box.
- Protect your feet from trauma (stubbing a toe or pounding) by not going barefoot and wearing shoes that give your toes wiggle room in the toe box.

Neuromas

A neuroma is a benign growth that "pinches" nerves between the third and fourth toes, according to the Canadian Podiatric Medical Association. It is also called Morton's neuroma. The possible causes are biomechanical deformities, trauma, shoes that cause the toes to be squeezed, heredity, and high-heeled shoes, which can increase pressure on the forefoot.

Symptoms

Nueroma symptoms include:
- Pain in the forefoot and between the toes
- Tingling and numbness in the ball of the foot
- Swelling between the toes
- Pain in the ball of the foot when weight is placed on it

Treatment

Wear shoes with room for the toes to move and thick shock-absorbent soles. Avoid shoes with heels higher than two inches. Resting your foot and massaging the affected area can provide temporary relief, and wearing over-the-counter shoe pads can relieve the pressure.

If left untreated, neuromas tend to get worse. If a neuroma is underdeveloped, thick-soled shoes with a wide toe box may be all you need to resolve the problem. Padding and taping at the ball of the foot may change the abnormal function and relieve the symptoms.

Anti-inflammatory drugs and cortisone injections can ease pain and reduce inflammation. Custom shoe orthotics can improve foot function. If everything else fails, surgery removes the inflamed nerve.

Prevention

Best steps to prevent neuromas:
- Wear shoes (and especially exercise shoes) with adequate room in the front to prevent compressing the toes.

Morton's neuroma

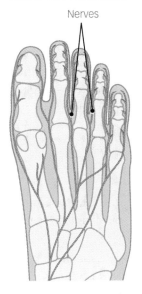 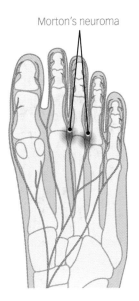 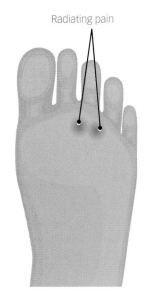

Nerves   Morton's neuroma   Radiating pain

© Aksana Kulchytskaya - Dreamstime

Pain from Morton's neuroma radiates from "pinched nerves" between the bones of the third and fourth toes.

- Wear shoes that have padding under the ball of the foot.
- Avoid prolonged time in shoes with a narrow toe box or excessive heel height.

Lupus

Lupus is a disease that causes the immune system to attack healthy areas of the body. A frequent symptom is inflamed and achy joints, including those in the feet and ankles. One survey found that achy joints were reported in 95 percent of Lupus cases.

The disease affects women 10 to 15 times more often than men, usually develops between the ages of 15 and 44, and is two to three times more common among African Americans, Hispanics, and Native Americans than among whites.

Patients with lupus can experience swelling and pain in their feet and ankles as a side effect of the disease. "Lupus foot" in particular is a deformity of toes and joints that can lead to pain when walking. Excess fluid from kidney failure can lead to more swelling in the lower extremities.

The American College of Rheumatology

suggests that if a patient has four or more conditions on a list of 11 criteria, that person is assumed to have lupus. The list includes the facial rash, photosensitivity, ulcers in the mouth, kidney dysfunction, and the presence of various blood components. Lupus is misdiagnosed about 15 percent of the time, and there is no single lab test that can determine whether a person has the condition.

Treatment

Once lupus is diagnosed, treatment falls into drug and non-drug categories. Medications include nonsteroidal anti-inflammatories, acetaminophen, steroids, anti-malaria drugs, and drugs that support the immune system.

Non-pharmacologic treatment strategies are 1) defense against the sun, 2) exercise to protect against disease, obesity, and osteoporosis, and 3) dietary measures, in some cases. Certain foods (alfalfa seeds, for example) may trigger lupus symptoms, while others (vitamins, minerals, and omega-3 fatty acids found in foods such as fatty fish and plant-based oils) are associated with improved symptoms of lupus.

Other ways of relieving symptoms are to elevate your feet when possible, wear shoes with a wider fit, try massages and warm baths, and wear compression socks or support pantyhose. Exercise can improve circulation.

Peripheral Artery Disease

Peripheral artery disease (PAD) is a narrowing of the arteries in the legs, stomach, arms, and head, according to the American Heart Association (AHA). It is most commonly seen in the legs.

PAD affects 8 to 12 million Americans, and most of them are over the age of 50. It causes symptoms such as fatigue, pain in the feet and legs, foot pain that interferes with sleep, and wounds or ulcers that are slow to heal.

People with high blood pressure, diabetes, elevated cholesterol, and those who smoke are at greatest risk.

Treatment

Treatment focuses on reducing symptoms and preventing further progression of the disease. It includes:

- Medications to control blood pressure, prevent blood clots, and lower cholesterol
- Physical therapy to increase strength and improve circulation
- Dietary changes to lower cholesterol and manage weight
- Smoking cessation
- Surgery to unblock, open, or bypass blocked arteries

The AHA says that regular physical activity is an effective treatment for PAD symptoms. Walking and leg exercises can ease symptoms, but should be approved by your doctor and performed under the direction of a physical therapist.

When conservative treatments are

Angioplasty for Peripheral Artery Disease

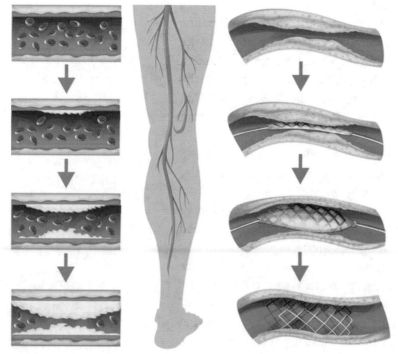

© Aksana © Blueringmedia | Dreamstime

Foot pain could be related to peripheral artery disease (PAD). An angioplasty and stent replacement is a common treatment for PAD.

ineffective, minimally invasive surgery may be recommended. Angioplasty and stent replacement are examples of those procedures.

Plantar Warts

Plantar warts are small growths on the skin caused by a virus. There are two types, according to the American College of Foot and Ankle Surgeons (ACFAS). A solitary wart is a single wart that often increases and may eventually multiply. Mosaic warts are a cluster of several small warts growing closely together. They are more difficult to treat than solitary warts. Plantar warts are caused by direct contact with the human papillomavirus (HPV).

Symptoms

Plantar wart symptoms include:

- Thickened skin that resembles a callus
- Pain when walking or standing
- Tiny black dots (actually dried blood contained in capillaries) on the surface of the wart

Treatment

Plantar warts may clear up without treatment, but most patients don't want to wait. The goal is to remove the wart or warts. That can be done with topical or oral medications, laser therapy, cryotherapy, acid treatments, or surgery.

The ACFAS warns people not to try to remove warts themselves. Folk remedies—and there are many of them—remain unproven and may be dangerous. Seek a podiatrist or dermatologist.

Prevention

The Mayo Clinic says that you can reduce your risk of plantar warts if you avoid direct contact with warts (including your own), keep your feet clean and dry, and avoid walking barefoot around swimming pools and locker rooms.

Don't pick or scratch warts and don't use the same emery board, pumice stone,

10 Tips for Healthy Feet

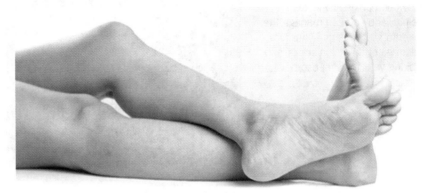

© Ziprashantzi | Dreamstime

Most of the problems described in this chapter can be avoided. Below are tips for maintaining healthy feet.

- Inspect your feet regularly.
- Maintain good foot hygiene.
- Hydrate the skin with lotions or creams.
- Cut toenails straight across.
- Avoid walking barefoot.
- Exercise—even by just walking—every day.
- Alternate shoes daily so they can dry out.
- Buy shoes that are comfortable and won't require a "breaking in" period.
- Buy shoes later in the day when your feet have expanded.
- Avoid pointed-toe styles and high heels.

or nail clipper on warts as you use on your healthy skin and nails.

Stone Bruises

A stone bruise is a painful, inflammatory condition on the bottom, forefoot area (the ball of the foot). It could be caused by an injury, overuse, or a structural defect.

The pain increases over time and usually becomes noticeable when walking. It is typically described as a burning or stabbing sensation. More pain is felt when the toes are pulled upward or when the joints are pressed.

Home treatment includes rest, ice, compression, and elevation (RICE). Changing shoes might help, especially for women who wear high heels.

If symptoms don't subside within a week, contact your primary care physician or a podiatrist. Most doctors will recommend limiting activity when a bone bruise is near a joint and giving the injury time to heal.

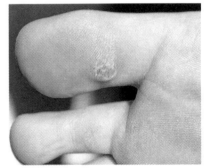

© Andrei Zakharov | Dreamstime

The skin of a plantar wart, thick and hard, can cause pain when simply walking or standing.

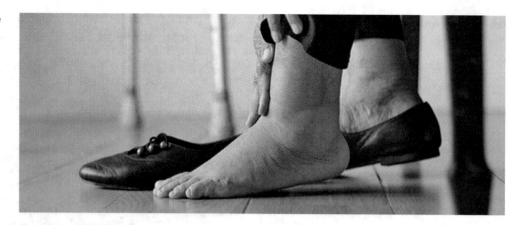

You can ease the problem of swollen ankles by losing weight, and you can manage the condition by elevating your feet, wearing compression socks, and soaking your feet in Epsom salts.

Swollen Ankles

Swollen ankles and feet are uncomfortable, but not generally an emergency—although they do merit medical attention (they can indicate serious diseases in the heart, kidney, or liver). The condition happens when the body retains fluid in the lower legs, ankles, and feet. Both feet are usually affected simultaneously.

Swollen feet are usually a symptom of something else, but if other diseases are ruled out, they can be managed by wearing compression socks, elevating your feet, flexing and extending your ankles, losing weight, and soaking your feet and ankles in a cool bath filled with Epsom salt.

Adding 200 to 400 milligrams of magnesium to your diet may limit water retention. Foods highest in magnesium include leafy greens, nuts, seeds, whole grains, legumes, avocados, bananas, and some fatty fish.

For best results, use more than one therapy at a time (compression socks after exercise, for example).

Toenail Fungus

The medical term for toenail fungus—onychomycosis—is not anymore pleasant to hear or see than the condition itself. The infection is common, easy to get (present in 20 percent of adults 60 and over), begins with a white or yellow tip of the toenail, and can spread to other nails. An affected nail can thicken, separate from the skin beneath, or crumble.

One other warning: Toenail fungus can last a lifetime.

Merely walking barefoot in the same area where someone with toenail fungus has walked is enough to get the infection. Wearing sweaty shoes, socks, or boots creates the perfect environment for the fungus to exist.

Treatment

Early diagnosis and treatment can prevent the fungus from spreading to other parts of your body and to other people, according to the American Academy of Dermatology. It is treated by topical solutions like Penlac, Jublia, and Kerydin, but there are no guarantees that they will work, and they must be used for months to have an effect.

Oral prescription medications are effective 50 to 75 percent of the time, and they have to be taken for at least nine months and up to a year. These medications have higher cure rates than topical solutions. They include the products Fulvicin, Lamisil, Sporanox, and Diflucan.

The FDA has not approved any over-the-counter medications for toenail fungus.

Prevention

To prevent toenail fungus, take the same steps as you would to ward off athlete's foot. Here are some reminders:

- Avoid using shower floors, locker rooms, and athletic floors without foot protection (flip-flops, for example). Beware swimming pools as well.
- Don't wear tight shoes.

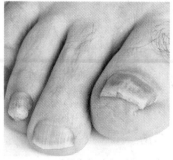

More than 20 percent of adults age 60 and over struggle with the problem of toenail fungus.

Swollen Feet May Require Prompt Medical Care

Take steps to see your physician if you have swollen feet: They could indicate a serious medical condition.

By Cindy Foley for University Health News

Swollen feet can be a normal inflammatory reaction due to overuse or a strain—the result of taking a bad step, for example. But swollen feet also can indicate a life-threatening medical condition, such as congestive heart failure. It's important to determine whether there's a known cause—like stepping in a hole—or if there are symptoms, like shortness of breath, in need of a physician's attention.

Ask yourself these questions: Has the swelling been ongoing (i.e., has it been there more than 24 hours)? Is the swelling worsening, and spreading up your leg, and are your feet getting bigger? Do you have other symptoms, such as fever, bruising, shortness of breath, dizziness, light-headedness, confusion, or pain? Is the swelling non-pitting—meaning you press on it for 10 or 15 seconds and the indentation doesn't stay?

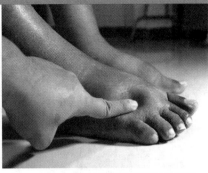

© Prot Tachapanit | Dreamstime

"Pitting" when pushing into your foot could be a sign of edema.

If you answered yes to any of these questions, you need to make a doctor's appointment. If you answered no to these questions but you're not certain why you're swelling, you still should talk with your doctor.

And if you also have symptoms like chest pain, shortness of breath, or dizziness, you need to get to an urgent-care facility or emergency room. Just four to six hours can make a difference in your heart health.

When Swollen Feet Are "Normal"

Sometimes swelling makes sense. Swelling is a natural component of inflammation—the redness, heat, and swelling is your body's first step in the healing process. And If you've been standing or walking for an unusual amount of time, some swelling is normal.

Swelling is an accumulation of fluid in the tissues—edema. Most swelling is "pitting," meaning you can press on it for 10 or 15 seconds and see the indent. An example of pitting edema is the indents our socks leave in our skin when we remove them. Some women experience "idiopathic"

(occuring without an underlying disease edema) during pre-menstruation or pre-menopause.

Non-pitting edema can be difficult to treat. It may indicate a problem with your lymphatic system or venous system. The swelling may be due to some type of internal pressure.

It's important not to blow off any type of swelling. According to a 2015 report from the European Society of Cardiology, one in five people will develop heart disease, but most people don't know that the main symptoms of heart failure are leg swelling (starting at the feet and moving up through the ankles) and becoming breathless, especially when lying down flat.

Red-Flag Swollen Feet

Bilateral swelling—both legs—often indicates a systemic cause, such as congestive heart failure. It also could be as simple as your body retaining water.

Unilateral swelling—one leg—is usually due to a localized problem like deep vein thrombosis, a blood clot, or lymph problem. These are dangerous conditions.

Swelling that increases dramatically over a short period of time, doesn't resolve in 24 hours, or doesn't improve with first aid warrants medical attention.

Any swelling that includes redness, blistering, or pain is not normal. Swelling that is great enough to make your shoes feel tight is not normal.

If you find you cannot walk comfortably, your feet also feel numb or "tingly," or your attempts at first aid do not bring improvement within 24 hours, you should seek medical attention.

If your swollen feet seemed to have occurred as you started a new medication, consult your doctor immediately.

Many life-threatening illnesses are associated with swollen feet, including:

- Allergic reactions
- Blood clots
- Cardiac disease
- Cellulitis
- Cervical cancer
- Congestive heart failure (CHF)
- Deep vein thrombosis (DVT)
- Hormonal imbalance
- Hypothyroidism
- Infections
- Kidney (renal) disease
- Liver (hepatic) disease, such as cirrhosis
- Lymphedema
- Obstructive sleep apnea
- Preeclampsia in pregnant women
- Pulmonary hypertension

These conditions warrant prompt medical attention. There are other symptoms related to these problems, but you may not be aware of the relationship. Don't take the chance.

Cindy Foley is a contributing editor at University Health News and executive editor of DogWatch and CatWatch, Belvoir Media Group publications produced with Cornell University.

Treating Swollen Feet: Applying first aid is an intelligent first step for swollen feet, especially if you're aware of the cause. Apply first aid in the form of PRICE:

P Protect the area.

R Rest your feet.

I Ice or a cold pack can help take down the swelling.

C Compress the area by properly applying a compression bandage

E Elevate your feet to a level where they are above your heart.

Some patients report massaging the swollen area helps reduce the severity. If you don't see improvement in 24 hours, consult your physician.

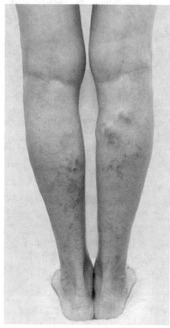

© Solarisys13 | Dreamstime

There are simple measures you can take to slow the progression of varicose veins: Don't sit cross-legged, don't stand for long periods of time, and don't smoke—and do make sure you get regular exercise.

What's Next?

Chapter 4 is about preventing foot and ankle problems with suggestions regarding shoes, socks, slippers, hygiene, nutrition, and exercise.

- Nail polish and acrylic nails make them more susceptible to infection.
- Keep your feet as clean and dry as possible, especially between the toes.

Varicose Veins

Varicose veins affect one in five adults and half of people over the age of 50 in the U.S. Although they are an indication of weak or damaged veins, they are usually more of a cosmetic problem than one that requires medical attention.

Muscles push blood back toward the heart through veins. Veins have valves that prevent blood from backing up in your legs or pooling in your ankles. When the valves are compromised, the result is varicose veins.

They can be blue, purple, red, bulging, gnarly, swollen, bumpy, enlarged, twisted, and snakelike. Spider veins indicate the same problem on a smaller scale. Clusters of veins close to the surface of the skin are red, blue, or purple, and can appear on the face or legs.

Risk Factors

- Age
- Genetic predisposition
- Pregnancy
- Hormonal changes
- Obesity
- Exposure to sun
- Sitting with legs crossed
- Standing for long periods of time

Symptoms

Pain in the legs can get worse when sitting or standing for long periods of time. Other symptoms are cramping, throbbing, a heavy leg feeling, itchy skin, darkening skin, and restless leg syndrome.

They also may lead to more dangerous conditions, including deep vein thrombosis, which is a blood clot in a deeper vein.

Treatment

Sclerotherapy is a non-surgical treatment for spider veins in which a chemical irritant is injected into a vein, which causes it to collapse and dry out.

Foam sclerotherapy involves injection of a foam solution into larger varicose veins to close them off.

Laser surgery sends surges of concentrated light into a vein to collapse it.

Ambulatory phlebectomy is an older technology in which the vein is removed through small incisions in the skin. It is not recommended for patients unable to walk on their own or those who wear compression stockings.

In advanced cases, endoscopic vein surgery is performed. A small incision is made and a surgical device at the end of a camera closes the vein. Usually this is same-day procedure and can be performed by an interventional radiologist.

Prevention

The single most important thing you can do to slow down the development of new varicose veins is to wear compression support stockings, according to the U.S. Office of Women's Health. Other measures include:

- Limiting sun exposure
- Exercising regularly
- Maintaining a healthy weight—a body mass index under 25.0.
- Elevate your legs to prevent blood from pooling in lower extremities.
- Wearing lower-heeled shoes

Alternative Approaches

There are numerous anecdotal reports of apple cider vinegar as a treatment for varicose veins, but little supporting evidence in professional literature. Other home remedies that have been suggested are butcher's broom, grape leaves and seeds, horse chestnut, and sweet clover. None have been supported by compelling scientific evidence.

Prognosis

Varicose veins can be treated, and you may be able to prevent more varicose veins from developing by following common sense, healthy living rules.

Tread Carefully to Protect Diabetic Feet

Control your blood sugar, practice good self-care, and stay vigilant to avoid diabetic foot problems.

By Jim Black

The nervous system can be thought of like a tree, with the spinal cord as the trunk and the peripheral nerves of the feet as the tiniest branches. And, just as those miniscule limbs are easily broken by the elements, so too can the small nerves in the feet be damaged by diabetes.

This nerve damage, or neuropathy, and the loss of feeling that results from it are a key pathway that leads to diabetic foot complications, the worst of which being amputation.

The possible loss of sensation and circulation in your feet can cause major problems and put you at high risk of requiring an amputation, which is a major fear of people living with diabetes.

By controlling your blood sugar, protecting your feet, and working with your health-care team, you can take steps to protect your feet and avoid complications.

What You Can Do

If you have diabetes...

- Wash your feet daily, and dry them thoroughly, particularly in between your toes.
- Apply a moisturizing cream to the tops and bottoms of your feet, but not between your toes.
- Trim your toenails straight across.
- Wear socks and shoes whenever you're on your feet. Avoid going barefoot.
- Make sure your shoes fit well, and check the insides for any defects that could injure your feet.
- If your feet feel cold, wear warm socks. Do not warm your feet with electric blankets, hot water bottles, or heating pads.
- Promote blood flow to your feet by elevating them when you're sitting and not crossing your legs for extended periods. Move your toes and ankles up and down for five minutes, two to three times daily.

Diabetes and Your Feet

Poorly controlled diabetes can damage delicate nerve fibers and cause diabetic neuropathy, making it more difficult to sense injuries to the foot. Although neuropathy can develop at any time, it's more common in older adults and those who have had diabetes for a longer duration, with the greatest prevalence among people who have had diabetes for at least 25 years, according to the National Institutes of Health.

Many diabetes patients also have peripheral artery disease, or PAD, which reduces blood circulation to the legs, feet, arms, and other locations away from the heart. Inadequate blood flow limits your foot's ability to fight infection and heal from injuries. This combination of poor healing and an inability to sense injuries to the feet make people with diabetes more susceptible to foot ulcers and infections that could result in amputation.

Some of the hallmark signs of diabetic neuropathy and PAD in your feet include discoloration (you may notice that your feet appear darker), a decline in (or lack of) hair growth, skin changes (dry, peeling, cracking skin), feet that constantly feel cold, tingling/burning/numbness, and cramping.

Tell your doctor if you experience these symptoms. And, just as you should have your eyes checked annually if you have diabetes, undergo yearly foot exams to identify any signs of diabetic foot complications.

If you've been living with diabetes for more than 10 years, if you have a history of blood sugar levels that are not under control, or if your condition hasn't been treated for an extended period of time, you're at a higher risk of having diabetic foot problems.

Visit your doctor for a thorough foot exam every year, especially if you're over the age of 60.

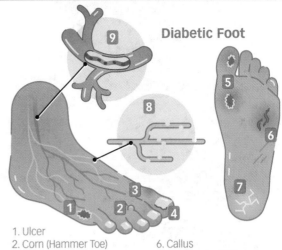

Diabetic Foot

1. Ulcer
2. Corn (Hammer Toe)
3. Bunion
4. Ingrown Toenails
5. Ulcers
6. Callus
7. Dry, Cracked Skin
8. Damaged Nerves
9. Reduced Blood Flow

© Wavebreakmedia Ltd | Dreamstime

Now that you know more about your feet and ankles and what types of ailments can befall them, you can take preventative action. This chapter is devoted to exercises that benefit the bones, muscles, ligaments, and tendons in your feet and ankles.

Prevention of Foot Issues

One key to preventing foot problems and other complications of diabetes is to manage your blood sugar carefully. Work with your health-care team to keep your blood sugar within the range your doctor recommends.

Inspect your feet daily, looking for sudden changes to skin color, red marks, swelling, cuts or breaks in the skin, or ingrown toenails. Keep an eye out for calluses. A common problem in diabetes patients, calluses can thicken, crack, and ulcerate.

You can help to control calluses by pumicing, but do so only after having a physical exam to gauge the sensitivity of your feet. Never cut away calluses or corns on your own without consulting your doctor.

Shielding your feet from harm is critical for preventing diabetic foot complications. That means wearing socks and shoes and not walking barefoot, whether you're in your home or outdoors. Accidents can happen, so keeping your feet protected can make a huge difference. Prevention is a better way to handle diabetic feet as opposed to fear.

Jim Black is executive editor of Men's Health Advisor, *a monthly publication produced by Belvoir Media Group in cooperation with Cleveland Clinic.*

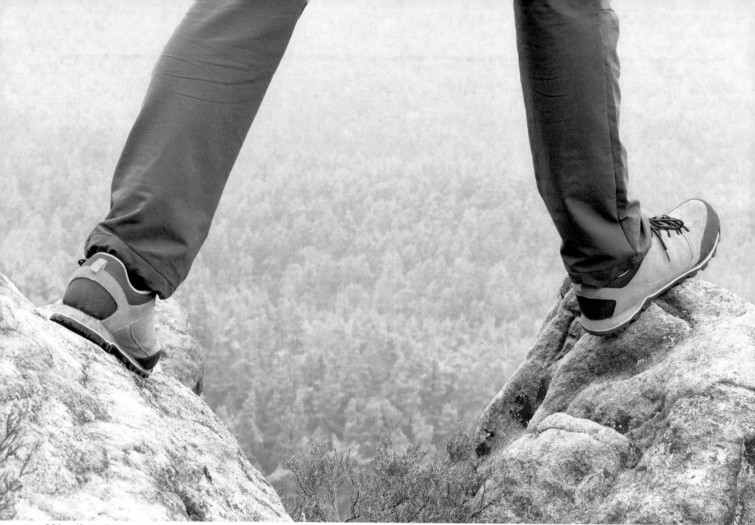

When our feet and ankles are pain-free, we tend to take them (and the mobility they give us) for granted. But don't forget your feet—follow the advice in this chapter to prevent issues from cropping up.

4 Preventing Foot and Ankle Problems

As with most medical issues, it's easier to prevent many foot and ankle problems than to treat them or live with them. As such, there are certain factors to keep in mind.

It helps if you wear the right kinds of shoes and socks, and keep your feet relatively clean.

And there is a stronger connection between diet and foot/ankle health than most would think. The link is direct for conditions like diabetes and inflammation, and indirect (but present) in others, such as osteoporosis and peripheral artery disease.

Then there's exercise and weight-loss, which ought to be near the top of the list for anyone serious about preventing foot and ankle problems.

But let's start with getting shoes that fit.

Shoes

You've no doubt bought shoes that just didn't fit right—and found yourself dealing with an annoying problem. Blisters. Corns. A callus. Maybe even an ankle sprain. So you likely appreciate the benefits of buying shoes that fit. As a reminder, here's our list of factors to keep in mind:

Factors That Affect Foot and Ankle Health

Don't shop early: Go shoe shopping in the afternoon or evening. Your feet naturally swell a bit (up to 8 percent) as the day wears on. Shoes that feel comfortable in the morning might feel tight later on. Wear the same type of socks to the store that you plan on wearing with the new shoes.

Get your feet measured for size: During middle age and beyond, get your feet re-measured every year. They tend to get larger and wider with age—at least one size, maybe more.

Get the right size: You don't have to know the exact shoe size when you shop. Know your approximate size based on shoes you already own, then look for fit and comfort. Each shoe manufacturer has its own shoe size standards. A size 9 shoe made by one company may be bigger or smaller than the same size in another brand. Trust your comfort level, not the size of a shoe. Consider tracing an outline of your foot and placing a shoe that you are considering on top of the outline. If they don't match, don't try them on.

Get the right length: Leave room for your feet to shift forward as you walk. There should about a half-inch between your longest (not your biggest) toe and the end of the shoe. Heels should fit snugly without pinching.

Get the right width: Look for shoes that are wider, not longer. For men's shoes, a narrow width is a B; a wide width is E. The average man wears a width-size D. Women's widths range from 4A (extra narrow) to 2E (extra wide). The average shoe width for women is B. If you have bunions, for example, you may benefit from wide toe box to avoid painful brushing of the shoe against the bump, which can cause pain and swelling throughout the day.

Shoes shouldn't have any space for your foot to move from side to side. They should be comfortably snug; not too tight or too loose. They should be wide enough so that the widest part of your foot (the ball of the foot) is comfortable. They should also provide a comfortable degree of arch support.

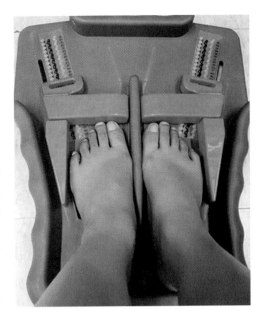

© Piyamas Dulmunsumphu | Dreamstime

It pays to do it right: When shopping for shoes, make sure the ones you pick out are the proper width for your feet. And take them for a "test drive"—a walk around the store can tell you whether you've got a good fit.

If you're still having a shoe size problem, try another brand instead of another size.

Buy for the bigger foot: When one foot is larger than the other, buy shoes that fit the larger foot. You can make up for the extra space in the smaller foot with an insert or two pairs of socks.

Don't anticipate "break-in" time: There should be no break-in time for new shoes; they should feel comfortable the first time you put them on.

Try them out: When buying new shows, walk around the store on at least two different surfaces (carpet and hard floor, for

NEW FINDING

High-Heel Shoes: Are Their Psychological Benefits to Women Worth the Health Risks?

Researchers in England reviewed 47 studies on the use of high-heel shoes and their effect on gender identity, attractiveness, and foot/ankle health. The review provided clear evidence of an association between high heels and bunions, musculoskeletal pain, osteoarthritis, and injuries, but a positive effect on perceived attractiveness and attitudes of the opposite gender. The authors concluded that it is important to respect a person's freedom of footwear choice, but that potential foot and ankle issues related to high heels should be recognized and addressed.

BMC Public Health, Aug. 1, 2017

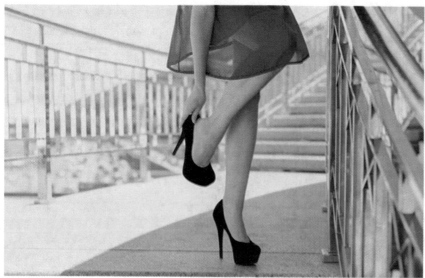
© Yelizaveta Tomashevska | Dreamstime

Being fashionable has its drawbacks—especially from the perspective of your feet.

example) to get a good feel. Take them off, put them on again, and take another lap. A test drive or two will make your decision easier.

Don't be a slave to fashion: Avoid shoes that are pointed because they crowd the toes. Women should avoid high heels in general because they put too much pressure on the forefoot. Long-term use of high heels can contribute to backaches, knee pain, and sprained ankles.

Be smart with online buys: If you shop for shoes online, ask about the return policy. Many companies are offering lenient terms and even encouraging customers to buy two pairs (with different sizes) to see which is better. Make sure the company will pay for return shipping.

More Than Style

Getting the right-fitting shoe is about more than comfort and style. It's about potential foot and toe-related problems that

---

You May Have Aging Feet If . . .

- You're having more regular aches and pains.
- Your feet are developing bunions.
- Your toes are showing signs of "clawing" (digging into the soles of your shoes).
- You are having circulatory problems such as varicose or spider veins.

---

send 7 million Americans to the doctor every year. Look for value, quality, and a good fit. You can get all three in one pair of shoes. A good shoe is a good investment for your foot and ankle health. Don't let a few dollars keep you from making the right choice.

Footwear for Aging Feet

Older adults have more foot and ankle problems than younger adults, and there are specific features that are important in shoes for older adults.

Some footwear tips:

- Resist the urge to wear slippers around the house. They can make things worse because they encourage or force you to shuffle rather than letting joints work as they should.
- Avoid plastic, easy-to-clean shoes that don't allow your feet to breathe and don't stretch to accommodate your foot size.
- Look for shoes that have cushioning or shock-absorbing soles that are comfortable while walking.
- Get a pair of shoes that keep the heel firmly in place but that you can take off easily.
- Lace, strap, buckle, or Velcro fastening shoes provide more support than a slip-on.
- Make sure your shoes are roomy enough when your feet swell.

Shoe Inserts and Orthotics

Shoes inserts are over-the-counter products. Orthotics are prescribed by a doctor and designed for your specific foot, says the American Podiatric Medical Association. Shoe inserts can cushion your feet, provide comfort, and support the arches, but they can't correct mechanical foot problems or cure long-standing foot issues.

Both inserts and orthotics can be helpful, but ask your doctor if one of them might be better for your feet.

Shoe Insole Sensors May Promote Safe Walking, Protect Against Falls

Researchers at Victoria University in Australia say that new insole sensor technologies have the potential to enhance the effectiveness of shoe insoles. Shoe insole additions or modifications improve ankle joint support, absorb shock, improve reaction speed, and help maintain balance. Insole sensor technology, such as in-shoe pressure management and motion capture systems, will make it possible to precisely monitor gait, allowing patients and doctors to observe how shoe insoles change walking patterns. Integration of wearable sensors into shoe insoles will be a future direction for real-time gait measurement, safer walking, and protection against falls.

Sensors, May 8, 2018

The most common types of inserts are:

- Arch supports have an elevated feature that support the foot's natural arch.
- Heel liners, also called heel pads or heel cups, provide extra cushioning in the heel region.
- Foot cushions act as a barrier between your foot and your shoe to prevent rubbing against your heel or toes.
- Insoles slip into your shoes to provide extra cushioning and support.

Socks

Socks are as important as shoes, especially for middle-aged and older adults. Fit, durability, length, cushioning, type of material, and moisture management are features to consider.

Fit

Avoid socks that are too tight or too loose. Too-tight socks may constrict the toes; too-loose socks can wrinkle, pinch, and cause blisters. The height doesn't matter as long as it rises above the back of the shoe to prevent blisters. Don't buy socks that are shorter than the shoe.

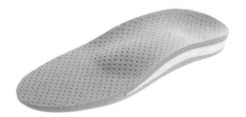

Shoe inserts or (as prescribed by a doctor) orthotics can make sure your feet are well supported.
© Yelizaveta Tomashevska | Dreamstime

Cushioning

A dense weave provides more padding, which can be helpful at the heel and ball of the foot. A cushioned heel also may last longer. Padded socks may be helpful for conditions such as plantar fasciitis and plantar warts. THORLO and OrthoFeet, among others, offer padded socks.

Material

"Moisture management" is the one area on which sock experts agree. Socks should have a wicking property to draw moisture (sweat) away from the foot so it can evaporate.

Socks made from 100 percent cotton absorb moisture and do not wick it away from the foot. They hold the moisture in and create a perfect environment for bacteria and fungi growth, which can lead to athlete's foot and foot odor. The moisture also can lead to blisters, calluses, and hot spots when combined with heat and friction.

Socks made out of synthetic fibers or cotton blends are ideal because they are durable, lightweight, and hug feet better.

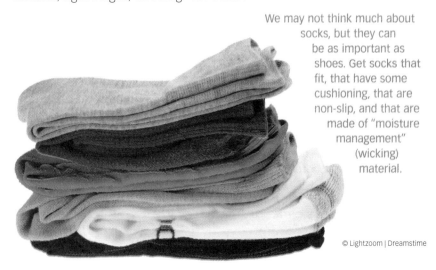

We may not think much about socks, but they can be as important as shoes. Get socks that fit, that have some cushioning, that are non-slip, and that are made of "moisture management" (wicking) material.

© Lightzoom | Dreamstime

Some have anatomical designs to ensure an optimal fit that reduces the risk of bunching in the shoe that can cause blisters or chafing. Synthetic fibers include the brands CoolMax and DryMax.

Non-Slip

Non-skid socks have rubber grips on the soles. A study in the *Journal of the American Podiatric Medical Association* found that, compared to standard socks, non-slip socks improved gait performance and may reduce the risk of slipping in older adults. Based on these findings, nonslip socks may be a safer footwear option than standard cotton socks for older people walking indoors on potentially slippery surfaces.

Compression Socks and Stockings

Compression socks are different from socks designed for diabetics. Compression socks are tightly knit and close-fitting to provide gentle pressure, improve circulation, and lower the risk of blood clots, according to *Berkeley Wellness*. However, compression socks do not have a universal standard for sizing. You'll have to find the right size for your foot and leg.

Those who might benefit are people who sit for long periods, have just had surgery, have varicose veins, spend a lot of time on their feet, or are more comfortable wearing them. There is little evidence that they improve athletic performance, even though some athletes and serious exercisers use them.

Some people should not wear compression stockings. They include patients with 1) peripheral neuropathy, 2) a skin infection, 3) a history of peripheral arterial bypass, 4) massive leg swelling, or 5) pulmonary edema. If you are not sure about wearing them, ask your doctor.

Over-the-counter (light) compression socks and stockings are widely available at retail pharmacies.

Socks for People with Diabetes

Diabetes socks are designed to protect the foot from injury, not to provide compression or improve circulation, according to *Diabetes Self-Management*. They should be soft, loose fitting, and provide padding on the sole of the foot.

Diabetes socks should fit the shape of the foot, ankle, and lower leg without wrinkles or bunching. They should be seamless or have flat seams to prevent irritation and non-binding tops to prevent cutting off circulation. As with any other good sock, diabetes socks should wick moisture away from the foot.

NEW FINDING

Indoor Footwear Types Can Affect Gait and Balance

Australian researchers studied the effects of two styles of footwear worn indoors on balance and gait patterns. Thirty women between the ages of 65 and 83 performed a series of tests wearing backless slippers with a soft sole vs. enclosed slippers with a firm sole and Velcro fastening.

Performances were best while wearing the enclosed slippers; the worst performances were with backless slippers. A majority of the women reported that they would consider wearing the enclosed slippers to reduce the risk of falling. The authors concluded that compared to backless slippers, indoor footwear with an enclosed heel, Velcro fastening, and a firm sole would be recommended to reduce the risk of falling.

Gerontology, February 2017

Avoid 100 percent cotton socks. They don't wick and are less durable than diabetic socks.

Slippers

Slippers are popular because they are easy to put on and take off, and they are comfortable. But they also can be dangerous. More than one study has shown many middle-aged and older adults have had a fall-related hip fracture while wearing slippers, and a recent study found that wearing backless indoor footwear carried a significantly higher risk of falls than enclosed slippers with a firm sole.

Below are some of the features to look for in safer slippers:

- Closed-in heels
- Velcro fasteners
- Hard, thin, non-slip soles
- Soft, comfortable insoles
- Light weight
- Adjustable fit

Hygiene

Clean feet means different things to different people. Podiatrists have pretty high standards of foot hygiene; they've seen what happens when people don't properly clean their feet.

Here are some of recommendations of podiatrists:

- Scrub your feet, including between your toes, every day. Use a soft sponge and soap.
- Change your socks daily and wear "breathable" footwear that wicks away perspiration.
- Keep your feet dry to prevent fungal foot infections. Without moisture, a fungus cannot survive.
- Dry your feet thoroughly, even between the toes, when you get out of the shower.
- Avoid sweaty feet by wearing moisture-wicking socks.
- Cut your toenails straight across. Nails that grow at angles can become ingrown toenails.

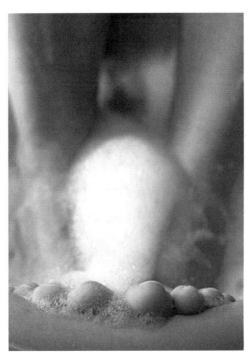

Keep your feet clean to prevent a variety of problems, including fungal foot infections.

- Examine your feet for problems.
- Protect your feet in public areas and surfaces.
- Don't share footwear.
- Don't hide discolored nails with polish. Let them breathe.
- Don't shave calluses. There are better ways to manage them.
- Address any foot health issues in their early stages. The longer you wait, the more difficult they are to heal.

Nutrition

Arthritis, peripheral artery disease, diabetes, osteoporosis, and obesity are conditions with a very clear connection with foot and ankle issues. (See "Tread Carefully to Protect Diabetic Feet" on page 55.)

Arthritis

Rheumatoid arthritis has been long recognized as an inflammatory disease, but there's a form of osteoarthritis that's clearly inflammatory as well, according to the Arthritis Foundation.

So-called inflammatory osteoarthritis, according to the Foundation, is "generally treated with nonsteroidal anti-inflammatory drugs and, very rarely, corticosteroid

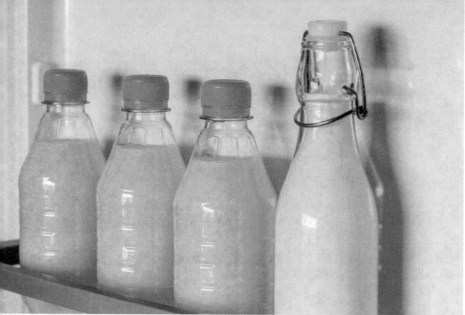
© Kanokphoto | Dreamstime

Eat a diet that defends against osteoporosis. That means getting calcium and vitamin D from such sources as fortified orange juice and dairy products, including milk or soymilk.

How Much Calcium Do You Need?	
AGE	AMOUNT
WOMEN	
50 and younger	1,000 mg/day (including food and supplements)
51 and older	1,200 mg/day
MEN	
70 and younger	1,000 mg/day (including food and supplements)
71 and older	1,200 mg/day

injections directly into the affected joints." The Foundation also says there are certain types of foods that reduce inflammation, as well as foods to limit or avoid.

Foods to Eat

- Fatty fish, such as salmon, tuna, sardines, and anchovies
- Berries, leafy greens, and cruciferous vegetables
- Nuts, including walnuts, pine nuts, pistachios, and almonds
- Legumes, including red beans, red kidney beans, and pinto beans
- Plant-based oils, especially olive oil
- Onions, carrots, and peppers
- Whole grains

Foods to Limit or Avoid

- Canned vegetables and soups (and other high-sodium, processed products)
- Salt (avoid or use in reduced amounts)
- Alcohol
- Red meat
- Fried foods
- Butter, shortening, lard

Peripheral Artery Disease (PAD)

Saturated fats, trans fat, and sodium increase the risk of peripheral artery disease, according to the American Heart Association. Limiting these foods decreases the risk.

Nutritional guidelines from the American Heart Association and American College of Cardiology recommend a diet high in oily fish (such as salmon, tuna, mackerel, and sardines) for individuals with cardiovascular disease, including PAD.

The *Journal of Vascular Disease* reported that consuming omega-3 foods is effective in lowering the risk of PAD. A *Journal of the American Heart Association* study concluded high-dose, short-duration fish oil supplementation improved serum triglycerides and had downstream benefits in patients with PAD.

Osteoporosis

Stress fractures associated with osteoporosis are frequently in the spine, but the feet and lower legs also are vulnerable, says the American Academy of Orthopaedic Surgeons. Getting enough calcium and vitamin D are ways to limit the damage or prevent it.

Calcium Sources

Food is the best source of calcium, says the National Osteoporosis Foundation: "Dairy products, such as low-fat and non-fat milk, yogurt, and (low-fat or fat-free) cheese (up to 1½ ounces daily) are high in calcium. Certain green vegetables and other foods contain calcium in smaller amounts."

Some juices, breakfast foods, soymilk, cereals, snacks, breads, and bottled water have calcium that has been added. If you drink soymilk or another liquid that is fortified with calcium, be sure to shake the container well because calcium can settle to

How Much Vitamin D Do You Need?	
WOMEN AND MEN	
AGE	**AMOUNT**
Under 50	400 to 800 IU/day
50 and older	800 to 1,000 IU/day

the bottom. And in fortified products, watch out for sodium content and added sugars.

Add calcium to many foods with a single tablespoon of nonfat powdered milk, which contains about 50 milligrams (mg) of calcium. Two to four tablespoons can be added to most recipes. "

Vitamin D Sources

Sunlight, food, and supplements are the best sources of vitamin D. The amount of vitamin D your skin makes depends on time of day, season, geographic latitude, and skin pigmentation. Depending on where you live, vitamin D production may decrease during the winter. Most people opt to get vitamin D from eating foods rich in vitamin D and taking vitamin D supplements.

Food sources of vitamin D are milk and other dairy products, fortified orange juice, soymilk, cereals, and "wild-caught" mackerel, salmon, and tuna.

Take vitamin D supplements only if you aren't getting enough from sunlight and food and if your doctor recommends it. Check to see if any other supplements you are already taking contain vitamin D and be sure to share with your doctor what you are taking. There are two types of vitamin D supplements—vitamin D2, synthetically made from plant life, and vitamin D3, which is the form your body makes when it converts sunlight to vitamin D. Vitamin D3 is the preferred form as it does a better job raising your vitamin D blood levels.

Obesity

Obesity compounds foot and ankle problems in several ways. The more weight the feet and ankles have to support, the more likely they are to sustain orthopaedic conditions like arthritis, not to mention high blood pressure, diabetes, and an elevated

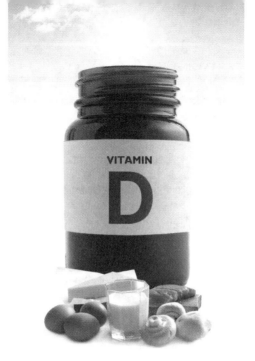

© Charlieaja | Dreamstime

Best sources of vitamin D: sunshine and D-rich foods (dairy products, fish, and mushrooms, for example) along with supplements as needed.

C-reactive protein level, which is a marker of inflammation. A 2018 *Journal of Pain* study found that people with a body mass index (BMI) of 30 or more were five times more likely to have plantar fasciitis than those with a BMI of 25.

Defined as a body mass index of 30 or higher, obesity is likely to result in physical inactivity—or maybe it's the other way around. It doesn't matter. Physical activity—as discussed in the next section—is critical for maintaining foot and ankle health.

BMI Categories

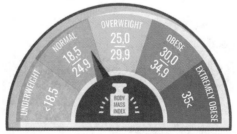

© Microvone | Dreamstime

Category	BMI
Underweight	Less than 18.5
Normal	18.5 to 24.9
Overweight	25 to 29.9
Obese	30 or higher

To find out your body mass index, use the BMI calculator at the National Heart, Lung, and Blood Institute's website. Visit nhlbi.nih.gov and type "BMI" in the search box.

Elevated Body Mass Index Strongly Associated with Plantar Fasciitis

The National Center for Complementary and Integrative Medicine conducted an analysis of data collected from 75,000 participants regarding the prevalence and treatment of plantar fasciitis pain. The data revealed that body mass index was strongly associated with the condition. Those with a BMI of 30 or more were five times more likely to have plantar fasciitis than those with a BMI less than 25. Among the other findings:

- 1 percent of U.S. adults reported a diagnosis of plantar fasciitis in the last year.

- The prevalence of plantar fasciitis was lowest in those between the ages of 18 and 44.

- The prevalence of plantar fasciitis was highest in those between the ages of 45 and 64.

- Those diagnosed by a medical specialist were twice as likely to use prescription medications for their condition than those diagnosed by a non-specialist.

Journal of Pain, March 27, 2018

Exercise

The last part of the foot and ankle health formula is exercise. Any exercise is better than no exercise at all, but we can narrow the options for you.

Start while sitting comfortably in your favorite chair or even lying in bed. Simple ankle rotations, extensions, and circles are examples of exercises good for flexibility and circulation. If you'd like something a bit more aggressive, standing calf raises and lunges are good for flexibility and strength. Chapter 5 illustrates those two exercises and 13 more.

If you really want to try something radical, go for a walk. For beginners, it doesn't have to be long or brisk. Start by walking around inside your home for five minutes, or to the end of the block and back, or on a treadmill, if you have access to one.

Walking is an activity in which you have complete control of the intensity level. Gradually increase the pace or time or distance or all three. Now you'll be getting some aerobic and muscular endurance mixed in with strength and flexibility.

Starter Program

Check the slightly modified version of the American College of Cardiology "Walking Program for Beginners" It's ambitious, but you can change the rules according to how you feel. Stay with the Week 1 program as long as you like or break up your walks into five- or 10-minute segments, two or three times a day.

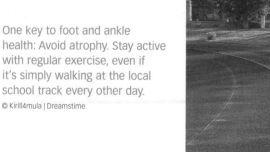

One key to foot and ankle health: Avoid atrophy. Stay active with regular exercise, even if it's simply walking at the local school track every other day.

© Kirill4mula | Dreamstime

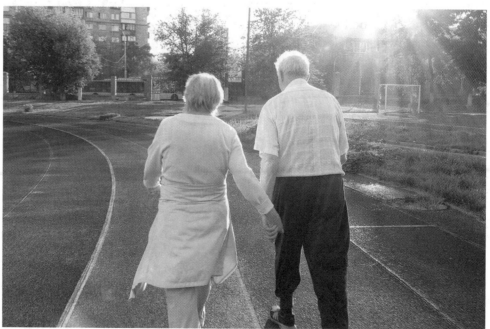

Walking Program for Beginners

WEEK	FREQUENCY	WARM-UP TIME	EXERCISE TIME	COOLDOWN TIME
1	Daily	5 minutes easy	5 minutes medium	5 minutes easy
2	Daily	5 minutes easy	8 minutes medium	5 minutes easy
3	Daily	5 to 7 minutes easy	11 minutes medium	5 minutes easy
4	Daily	5 to 7 minutes easy	15 minutes medium	5 minutes easy
5	Daily	5 to 7 minutes easy	20 minutes medium	5 minutes easy
6	5 times a week	10 minutes easy	25 minutes medium	5 minutes easy
7	5 times a week	10 minutes easy	30 minutes medium	5 minutes easy

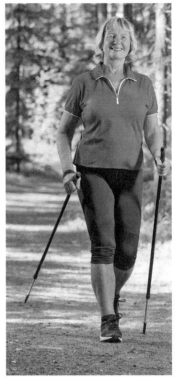

© Mikkolem | Dreamstime

Getting started on a daily or five-days-per-week walking routine will keep your feet moving and healthy. But that's not all: As noted at University Health News, walking at a moderate pace can lessen cancer risk, reduce mental decline, lower the chance of heart disease, improve joint function, reduce the risk of diabetes, and improve your energy level.

Sticking with It

The biggest single obstacle to an effective exercise program, whether for foot and ankle health or some other goal, is continuing with the program over an extended period of time—long enough to make a difference and a permanent part of your daily routine. Fifty percent of people who begin an exercise program drop out within six months.

Here are 10 suggestions to help you become a regular exerciser and to have healthy feet and ankles.

▶ **Set a goal.** Write it down. Make it measurable and observable. Set the bar low. Aim to under-promise and over-achieve:
I will walk _____*times a week*
for least _____*minutes*
for at least _____*weeks.*

▶ **Schedule it.** Don't wait until you have time.

▶ **Select a convenient location.** Closer is better.

▶ **Do it with a friend or group.** The evidence shows that you're more likely to adhere to an exercise program if you do it with others.

▶ **Make it enjoyable.** Listen to music or a podcast. Watch TV.

▶ **Exercise during commercial breaks.**

▶ **Track your progress.** Time, distance, speed, repetitions, whatever you can measure.

▶ **Revise it,** if necessary. It's your program, so make it more or less challenging, depending on your specific situation. Anything to keep you going is okay.

▶ **Don't give up if you miss a day or two.** It happens to everyone. Just pick up and get going again.

▶ **Reward yourself,** but not necessarily with food.

What's Next?

Chapter 5 illustrates and provides instructions for 15 exercises that can improve foot and ankle circulation, strength, range of motion, and balance.

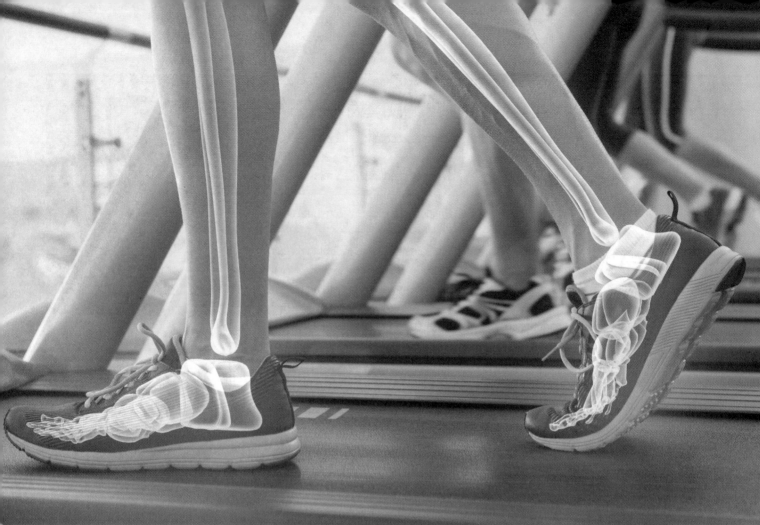

© Wavebreakmedia Ltd | Dreamstime

Now that you know more about your feet and ankles and what types of ailments can befall them, you can take preventative action. This chapter is devoted to exercises that benefit the bones, muscles, ligaments, and tendons in your feet and ankles.

5 Easy Exercises for Foot and Ankle Health

The 15 exercises illustrated in this final chapter of *Foot & Ankle Health* are designed to increase circulation, range of motion, balance, strength, or a combination of all. Increase or decrease the difficulty by adjusting the:

- Number of repetitions (reps)
- Number of sets (the number of repetition cycles for any particular exercise performed during a single session)
- Intensity (amount of resistance)
- Frequency (number of days per week)
- Resting time between sets

With any exercise that's new to you, it's most sensible to begin with a low number of reps and sets, and then gradually move up. Don't overdo it. But don't be sporadic, either.

You can perform the flexibility exercises here on a daily basis. Perform the strength exercises on two to three nonconsecutive days per week to allow muscles and muscle groups to recover. Rest a minute or two between sets.

Each exercise has a number, name, purpose, illustration, and instructions. Most of them can be performed with little or no equipment, and all of them can be done at home or at a wellness center.

Exercises #5 and #6 require a resistance band. A resistance band is an inexpensive, strong, thin rubber band (Theraband is a commonly used commercial resistance band) that provides resistance for strengthening exercises.

Check with your doctor before beginning any vigorous or new exercise program.

TOES BACK

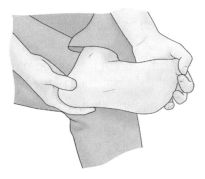

- Sit with one leg crossed over the other.
- Grasp your heel or ankle with one hand and your toes or ball of the foot in the other.
- Pull your toes up and back toward your shin.
- Hold for 10 to 30 seconds, relax, and repeat.
- Do 2 to 3 reps and 1 set.
- Change positions and pull the toes back on the other foot.

Variation: Complete the motion, hold for 1 to 3 seconds instead of holding for 10 to 30 seconds.

ANKLE FLEX/EXTEND

- In a seated position, extend your legs forward, heels on the floor.
- Flex both ankles, toes pointing up and toward your body.
- Hold for 10 to 30 seconds, relax, and repeat.
- Now extend your ankles, toes pointing down and away from your body, and hold for 10 to 30 seconds.
- Do 2 to 3 reps and 1 set.

Variation: Complete the motion, pause for 1–3 seconds instead of holding for 10–30 seconds.

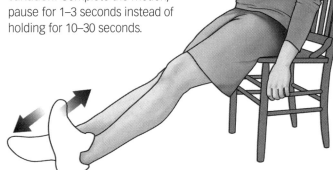

FOOT/ANKLE CIRCLES

- In a seated position, stretch your legs forward, heels on the floor.
- Lift one foot at a time (or both feet together) slightly off the floor, and make foot/ankle circles as large as possible.
- Do 10 to 20 circles, stopping halfway through to change directions.
- Do 1 set.

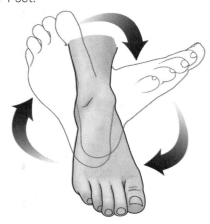

LOWER LEG TOWEL STRETCH

- Sit on the floor with one or both legs extended in front.
- Wrap a towel around the bottom of one foot, holding each end of the towel in your right and left hands, respectively.
- Pull back on the towel, flexing your ankle so that the top of your foot moves toward your body.
  - Don't bend your knee.
  - Hold for 20 to 30 seconds, relax, and repeat for a total of 2 to 3 repetitions.
  - Do 2 to 3 sets.
  - Change positions and pull the towel back on the opposite foot.

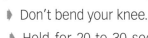

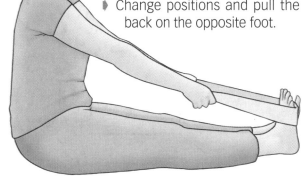

ANKLE INVERSION

▶ Secure one end of a resistance band to a table leg or sturdy object.

▶ Place the other end around the inside of your forefoot.

▶ Keep the heel still and move your forefoot inward, pulling against the band.

▶ Relax and return to the starting position.

▶ Do 5 to 10 reps and 1 set.

▶ Switch feet and repeat.

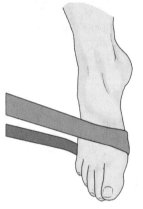

ANKLE EVERSION

▶ Place a resistance band around the outside of your forefoot.

▶ Keep the heel still and move your forefoot to the outside against the resistance of the band.

▶ Relax and return to the starting position.

▶ Do 5 to 10 reps and 1 set.

▶ Switch feet and repeat.

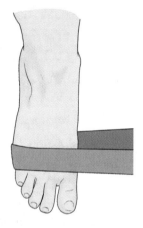

TOE RAISE/CALF RAISE

EXERCISE 7

▶ Stand near a secure object to hold onto for support.

▶ Feet parallel at shoulder width.

▶ Rise up on your toes to a point of resistance and hold for 10 seconds.

▶ Return to the starting position and repeat the movement.

▶ Work up to 8 to 10 reps and 2 to 3 sets.

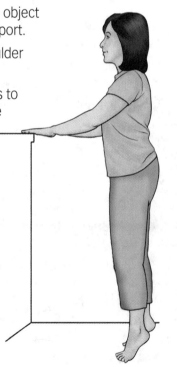

STAIRSTEP CALF RAISE

EXERCISE 8

▶ Stand on a stairstep, holding the handrail with one hand for support.

▶ Toes of both feet near the edge, heels below step level.

▶ Rise up on your toes and hold for 10 to 30 seconds.

▶ Slowly return to the starting position.

▶ Work up to 8 to 10 reps and 1 to 2 sets.

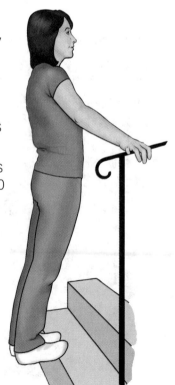

LUNGES

EXERCISE 9

- Stand with feet hip width apart.
- Take a long step forward (12 to 18 inches) with your right foot, keeping the heel of your back foot in contact with the floor.
- Don't extend the knee of your front foot past your toes.
- Hold for 2 to 3 seconds and repeat with the left foot forward.
- Work up to 8 to 10 reps (steps) and 1 set.

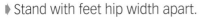

ACHILLES WALL STRETCH

EXERCISE 10

- Take a standing position facing a wall, both hands on the wall, one foot forward.
- Keep both feet flat on the floor as you lean forward.
- Hold for 20 to 30 seconds, relax, and return to the starting position.
- Do 2 to 3 repetitions and 1 set.
- Change positions and stretch the Achilles tendon of the opposite foot.

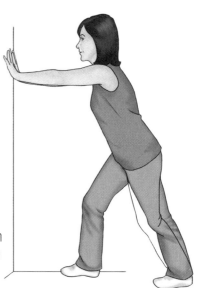

BALANCE WALK

EXERCISE 11

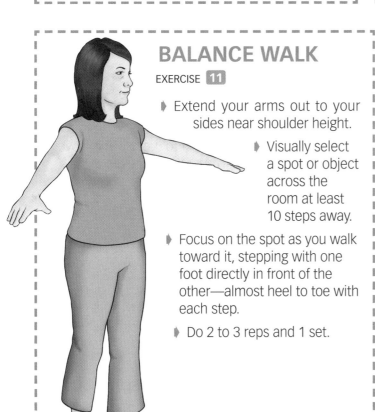

- Extend your arms out to your sides near shoulder height.
- Visually select a spot or object across the room at least 10 steps away.
- Focus on the spot as you walk toward it, stepping with one foot directly in front of the other—almost heel to toe with each step.
- Do 2 to 3 reps and 1 set.

WEIGHT SHIFT

EXERCISE 12

- Start from a standing position, back straight, shoulders back, feet slightly farther apart than your hips.
- Shift your weight from side to side, lifting your non-weight-bearing foot slightly.
- Balance for a few seconds every third (side) step.
- Continue for 30 to 60 seconds, then stop, rest, and repeat another 30 to 60 seconds. Do 1 set.

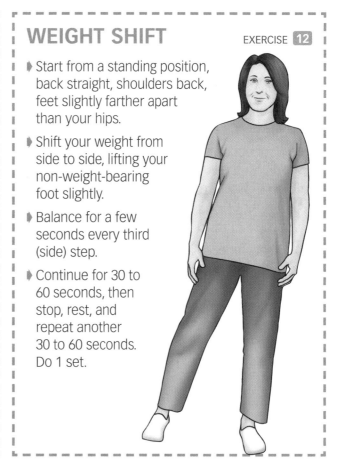

TOE WALKING, HEEL WALKING

EXERCISE 13

- ▶ Hold a rail or touch your hand against a wall for support, if needed.

- ▶ Walk forward on your toes, 10 to 20 steps, then walk 10 to 20 steps on your heels.

- ▶ Do 1 to 2 sets.

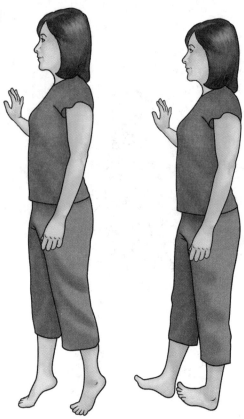

SINGLE LEG, TOWEL BALANCE

EXERCISE 14

- ▶ Fold a towel and place it on the floor.
- ▶ Stand on one leg with knee straight but not hyperextended.
- ▶ Lift your opposite foot slightly off the floor and hold your balance.
- ▶ Start at 15 seconds and work up to 1 minute.
- ▶ Do 3 sets for each leg.
- ▶ To decrease the difficulty, remove the towel and balance on each foot flat against the floor.

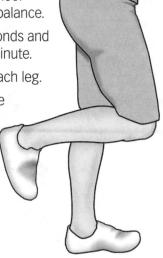

STANDING FOOT MASSAGE

EXERCISE 15

- ▶ Stand with a tennis ball under the arch of one foot.
- ▶ Slowly load your weight onto the ball and move your foot forward to apply pressure along the sole of your foot.
- ▶ Start at 30 seconds and work up to 3 minutes with each foot.
- ▶ Do 3 sets with both legs.
- ▶ To decrease the difficulty, perform the exercise from a seated position.

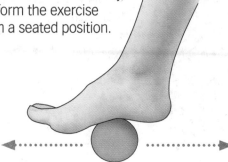

Achilles tendinitis: Inflammation of the tendon that connects the calf muscle to the heel.

acupuncture: Treatment based on the premise that a system of energy travels through medians in the body, and that stimulating pressure points along those medians can help heal the body.

alternative medicine: Non-mainstream practice used instead of conventional medicine.

athlete's foot: Fungal infection characterized by itching, burning, redness, and/or peeling.

bunions: Condition in which the joints of the big toe become deviated outward.

bursa: A fluid-filled sac that reduces friction in joints.

bursitis: Inflammation of the fluid-filled bursa sacs in joints.

callus: A thick layer of skin that develops, usually on the soles.

cartilage: Smooth material that covers the ends of long bones at the joints.

complementary medicine: Use of one or more non-mainstream practices in combination with conventional medicine.

compression socks: Tightly knit and close-fitting socks that provide gentle pressure to improve circulation.

computerized tomography (CT) scan: Computerized tomography images that provide detailed information about bones, blood, vessels, and soft tissue.

corn: Thick layer of outer skin that develops on a toe.

corticosteroids: Anti-inflammatory medications.

disease-modifying anti-rheumatic (arthritis) drugs (DMARDs): A class of medications used to slow down the disease process in rheumatoid arthritis.

fibromyalgia: A disorder marked by widespread musculoskeletal pain accompanied by fatigue, sleep, memory, and mood issues. Fibromyalgia, experts believe, may amplify sensations of pain by affecting our brain's processing of pain signals.

fibula: The smaller of the two bones in the lower leg.

gout: A type of arthritis characterized by needle-like crystals of uric acid in connective tissue.

integrative medicine: The practice of medicine in which complementary approaches are incorporated into mainstream care.

ligaments: Cord-like tissues that connect one bone to another.

joint capsule: The membrane sac that encloses joints.

Lupus: An autoimmune disease that often affects joints.

magnetic resonance imaging (MRI): An imaging technique that creates a 3-D image of soft tissues, connective tissue, and bones.

neuroma: Benign growth between the third and fourth toes, also called a pinched nerve.

non-steroidal anti-inflammatory drugs (NSAIDs): Medications—including aspirin, ibuprofen, naproxen, and others—that reduce pain, decrease fever, prevent blood clots, and (in higher doses) decrease inflammation.

obesity: A condition in which a person's body mass index (BMI) is greater than 30.

orthotics: Prescribed shoe inserts designed for a person's specific foot.

osteoarthritis: A common form of arthritis characterized by progressive degenerative changes in the cartilage of a joint.

osteoporosis: Progressive disease in which bones become thin, fragile, and at risk of fracture.

osteotomy: Surgery in which a damaged bone is cut or removed.

overweight: Condition in which a person's body mass index is 25 to 29.9.

orthopaedic surgeon: Medical doctor who treats the entire musculoskeletal system (including bones, joints, ligaments, muscles, nerves, and tendons).

peripheral artery disease (PAD): Narrowing of the arteries in the legs, stomach, arms, or head.

plantar fasciitis: Inflammation of the tissue that runs along the bottom of the foot from the heel to the base of the toes.

platelet-rich plasma (PRP): Patient's blood plasma that has been concentrated to produce 5 to 10 times more platelets than is typically found in blood.

podiatrist: Doctor of medicine who specializes in disorders of the foot and ankle.

Rest, Ice, Compression, Elevation (RICE): An acronym that describes the care and treatment of simple foot and ankle sprains, strains, and other injuries that cause swelling.

rheumatoid arthritis: Inflammatory disease thought to cause the body's immune system to attack the lining of the joints.

sesamoiditis: Inflammation of the sesamoiditis bones in the forefoot.

shoe inserts: Over-the-counter insert pads that provide comfort and arch support.

stem cell therapy: Technology that uses a person's own cells to grow or repair damaged tissue.

sprain: An injury caused by forcing a joint beyond its normal range of motion.

strain: A stretched or torn tendon or ligament.

tai chi: A martial art that combines relaxation, meditation, and deep breathing with continuous and structured exercises.

talus: The ankle bone.

tendinitis: Inflammation of the tendons, which connect muscles to bones.

tendons: Cords that connect muscles to bones.

therapeutic massage: Manipulation of muscle, connective tissue, tendons, and ligaments to enhance a person's health and well-being.

tibia: The shinbone.

varicose veins: An indication of weak or damaged veins characterized by swelling and blue, purple, or red veins close to the surface of the skin.

yoga: Type of exercise that incorporates movement, relaxation, and gentle breathing that may lead to improved balance and range of motion.

**American Academy of
Medical Acupuncture
(AAMA)**
medicalacupuncture.org
info@medicalacupuncture.org
310-379-8261
2512 Artesia Blvd., Suite 200
Redondo Beach, CA 90278

**American Academy of
Orthopaedic Surgeons
(AAOS)**
aaos.org
847-823-7186
9400 West Higgins Rd.
Rosemont, IL 60018-4262

**American Chiropractic
Association (ACA)**
acatoday.org
memberinfo@acatoday.org
703-276-8800
1701 Clarendon Blvd., Suite 200
Arlington, VA 22209

**American College
of Foot and Ankle
Surgeons (ACFAS)**
acfas.org
info@acfas.org
800-421-2237
8725 West Higgins Rd.
Chicago, IL 60631

**American Council
on Exercise**
acefitness.org
support@acefitness.org
888-825-3636
4851 Paramount Dr.
San Diego, CA 92123

**American Fibromyalgia
Syndrome Association
(AFSA)**
afsafund.org
kthorson@afsafund.org
520-733-1570
P.O. Box 32698
Tucson, AZ 85751

**American Podiatric
Medical Association (APMA)**
apma.org
844-571-4357
9312 Old Georgetown Rd.
Bethesda, MD 20814

Arthritis Foundation
arthritis.org
844-571-4357
1355 Peachtree Street N.E.,
6th Floor
Atlanta, GA 30309

**Centers for Disease
Control and Prevention**
cdc.gov
800-232-4636
1600 Clifton Rd.
Atlanta, GA 30329-4027

Lupus Foundation of America
lupus.org
info@lupus.org
888-558-0121
2121 K Street NW, Suite 200
Washington, DC 20037

**National Center for
Complementary and
Integrative Health**
nccih.nih.gov
info@nccih.nih.gov
888-644-6226
9000 Rockville Pike (NCCIH)
Bethesda, MD 20892

**National Fibromyalgia
& Chronic Pain Association**
fmcpaware.org
info@fmcpaware.org
801-200-3627
31 Federal Ave.
Logan, UT 84321

National Council on Aging
ncoa.org
571-527-3900
251 18th St. S, Suite 500
Arlington, VA 22202

**National Heart, Lung,
and Blood Institute**
nhlbi.nih.gov
nhlbiinfo@nhlbi.nih.gov
301-592-8573
Bldg 31, Rm 5A52
31 Center Dr. MSC
Bethesda, MD 20892

**National Osteoporosis
Foundation**
nof.org
800-231-4222
251 18th St. S, Suite 630
Arlington, VA 22202

**U.S. Food & Drug
Administration**
fda.gov
888-463-6332
10903 New Hampshire Ave.
Silver Spring, MD 20993

**U.S. National Library
of Medicine**
medlineplus.gov
8600 Rockville Pike
Bethesda, MD 20894

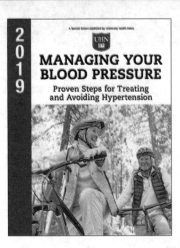
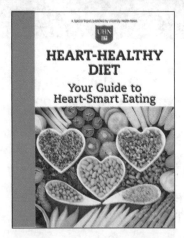
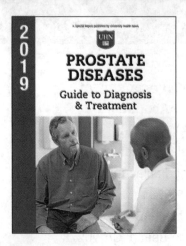
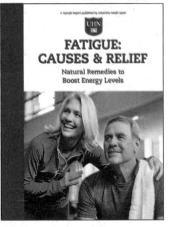
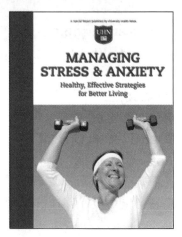
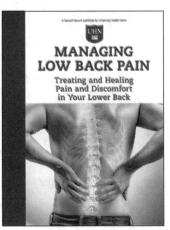
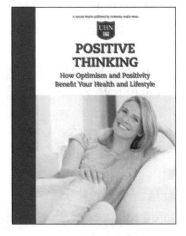
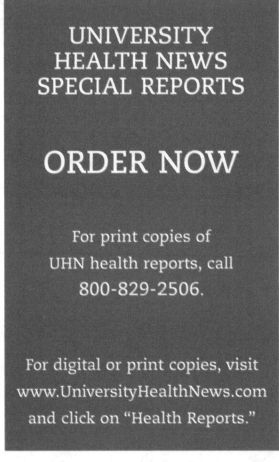
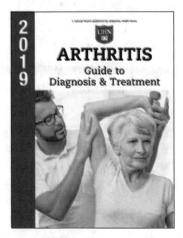
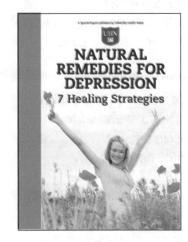
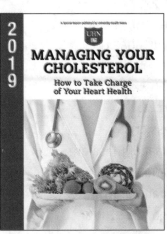